Leadership Skills for Dental Professionals

Leadership Skills for Dental Professionals

Begin Well to Finish Well

Raman Bedi, BDS, MSc, DDS, hon DSc, DHL, FDSRCS (Edin), FDRCS (Eng), FFGDP, hon FDSRCS (Glas), hon FFPH
Emeritus Professor, King's College London, England, UK
Honorary Chair, University of Western Cape, Cape Town, South Africa
Former Chief Dental Officer, England, UK

Andrew Munro, MA, C Psychol, AFBPS
Director, Envisia Learning
Cambourne, England

Mark Keane, MA, PPABP
Director, Favorly
Scotland, UK

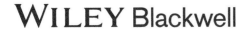

WILEY Blackwell

This first edition first published 2022
© 2022 John Wiley & Sons Ltd

Registered Offices
John Wiley & Sons, Inc., 111 River Street, Hoboken, NJ 07030, USA
John Wiley & Sons Ltd, The Atrium, Southern Gate, Chichester, West Sussex, PO19 8SQ, UK

Editorial Office
The Atrium, Southern Gate, Chichester, West Sussex, PO19 8SQ, UK

For details of our global editorial offices, customer services, and more information about Wiley products visit us at www.wiley.com.

Wiley also publishes its books in a variety of electronic formats and by print-on-demand. Some content that appears in standard print versions of this book may not be available in other formats.

Library of Congress Cataloging-in-Publication Data

Names: Bedi, Raman, author. | Munro, Andrew (Chartered psychologist),
   author. | Keane, Mark, author.
Title: Leadership skills for dental professionals : begin well to finish
   well / Raman Bedi, Andrew Munro, Mark Keane.
Description: Hoboken, NJ : Wiley-Blackwell, 2022. | Includes
   bibliographical references and index.
Identifiers: LCCN 2022013673 (print) | LCCN 2022013674 (ebook) | ISBN
   9781119870098 (paperback) | ISBN 9781119870104 (adobe pdf) | ISBN
   9781119870111 (epub)
Subjects: MESH: Dentistry | Leadership
Classification: LCC RK61 (print) | LCC RK61 (ebook) | NLM WU 21 | DDC
   617.6–dc23/eng/20220610
LC record available at https://lccn.loc.gov/2022013673
LC ebook record available at https://lccn.loc.gov/2022013674

Cover Design: Wiley
Cover Image: © andresr/Getty Images

Set in 9.5/12.5pt STIXTwoText by Straive, Pondicherry, India
Printed and bound by CPI Group (UK) Ltd, Croydon, CR0 4YY

C9781119870098_290722

This book is dedicated to my parents, Satya Pal and Raj Bedi

Contents

Preface

I remember attending the Colgate-Palmolive 200th anniversary celebration at the New York Stock Exchange in 2006, and meeting Raman Bedi for the first time as he joined Colgate-Palmolive's CEO to ring the trading bell. When we later met in London, Raman shared with me his vision of improving children's oral health for the world's most disadvantaged, and his thoughts on why this would require a different approach to leadership. In all honesty, I wondered how realizing this powerful vision could be possible. It was from this conversation that the Senior Dental Leadership (SDL) programme was born: a public-private collaboration between two prestigious academic institutions, King's College London and Harvard University, and two healthcare corporations, Henry Schein and Colgate-Palmolive.

Now, almost 14 years later, the SDL programme has gone from strength to strength, with more than 200 alumni from 47 countries working in innovative and imaginative ways to provide access to care to children in need in their countries.

In truth, no individual is born a leader. Although some may associate leadership with a range of skills and operating styles, for the most part, leadership is the accumulation of "good habits," built and strengthened over time as each of us encounter various opportunities and challenges in our personal and professional lives. This book is a guide for the dental professional who strives to become a more efficient and effective leader who fosters an environment where her or his patients and colleagues thrive and makes a positive difference in the wider community.

It has been truly extraordinary to see the tremendous impact that the SDL programme has had on the dental profession over the past 14 years, and, in turn, the positive impact these professionals have had on improving children's oral health around the world. This book builds on the principles of leadership that have fueled the success of SDL to help ensure that leadership – personal and professional – will continue to thrive in the dental profession as a whole.

Stanley M. Bergman
Chairman of the Board and CEO
Henry Schein, Inc.

Testimonials

USA

Harvard University has an illustrious history in training individuals from all walks of life. Through our collaboration with the Senior Dental Leaders Programmes, we can upscale our work in the dental field. I am excited about the possibilities this collaboration can bring and the improvements we can expect in the oral health of our global society. This book will help in that endeavour.

Professor Bruce Donoff, Former Dean, Harvard School of Dental Medicine

Brazil

The changing face of modern dentistry in Brazil requires strong and effective leadership for the provision of optimal dental care, health promotion and building partnerships with other professions. This book provides dentists with strong multidisciplinary skills, enabling them to combine clinical dentistry with leadership knowledge.

The Certificate in Advanced Dental Leadership provided unique and high-level guidance to young Brazilian dentists for shaping their careers, contributing to the dental profession and helping people from disadvantaged backgrounds. Now this book will also strengthen dentists' professional backgrounds, combining multidisciplinary clinical skills and leadership knowledge, and will build a network of next-generation dentists for Brazil.

Professor Sonia Groisman, Faculdade de Odontologia da UFRJ

Africa

Zambia's dental community needs leadership training and this book will help provide important leadership training. Leadership skills are important to my students as they are expected to take a central role in their provinces and districts after graduation in leading dental personnel and supporting staff.

Young dentists will also benefit with the training, as it is obvious that good leadership skills are a key to success. I believe the earlier in a dental professional's career leadership skills are studied, developed, and harnessed, the better the individual will be able to effect change.

This book is a good initiative for Zambia. Our country has been lacking in dental leadership continuous professional development.

Dr Severine Nyerembe, Copperbelt University, Ndola Zambia

This is a very good book and it is very relevant for all the oral health professionals. Our School recently acquired a certificate of Registration as an Oral Health CPD provider in Rwanda, making it an easy opportunity for launching collaborative effort in CDEs and CPDs. Now this book will help our students to acquire the leadership skills that our country so badly needs.

Professor Muhumuza Ibra, Dean, School of Dentistry-College of Medicine and Health Science, University of Rwanda

China

I know that the Advanced Dental Leadership Programme is very useful for young dentists to develop their leadership skill, which is very important for their professional promotion, and now this book will also help in improving paediatric oral health in China. Therefore, on behalf of the Chinese Society of Paediatric Dentistry, I would like to express my warmest thanks to the Global Child Dental Fund and everyone involved.

Professor Man Qin, Professor of the department of Pediatric Dentistry, Peking University School and Hospital of Stomatology; Immediate past President of Chinese Society of Pediatric Dentistry; President of Pediatric Dentistry Association of Asia; Fellow of International College of Dentists

India

During the last decade the Global Child Dental Fund (GCDFund) has engaged and developed hundreds of the world's foremost dental health professionals through its unique Senior Dental Leaders Programme.

The need of the hour is to further strengthen the global dental community through enlightened leadership. In response to this challenge, this book will enable younger Indian dental professionals to hone their skills in dental leadership, innovation, creativity and effectiveness.

A true leader has the potential to translate vision into reality.

This book will foster an ecosystem for sharing and nurturing the best leadership practices within the dental fraternity. It will also be a vibrant platform for young dental practitioners to ideate on the future of our profession.

I invite you to embark on this journey of education and organisational discovery, so that together we can improve oral health services and reduce inequality around the world.

Professor Mahesh Verma, Director and former Principal, Maulana Azad Institute of Dental Sciences, and Vice-Chancellor, Guru Gobind Singh Indraprastha University

For senior-level dental leaders it has always been critical to instil in the next generation the importance of the pedagogy we have always worked to. This is to adapt to the needs of the hour to achieve optimum oral health for our fellow community members. This approach, born of deep care and concern, must always be at the nucleus of our profession.

The book is a much-needed opportunity for budding professionals to further their education and develop their dental leadership competencies. As senior dental leaders, we promise to walk with you as you educate and empower yourselves to tackle the pressing challenges in global oral health.

Professor Satyawan G. Damle, Ex Dean Nair Hospital Dental College Mumbai & Ex Vice Chancellor Maharishi Markandeshwar University, Mullana. Ambala, India

The future of the dental profession must be in the hands of dentists possessing superior leadership skills. The next-generation dentistry demands effective, efficient leadership for several tasks including the delivery of optimal dental care, building partnerships with other professions, and health promotion. This book provides training and imparts state-of-the art guidance to dental students for shaping their careers and contributing to the profession and caring for the most disadvantaged people in our societies.

Professor Ashwin M. Jawdekar, Professor and Head, Department of Paediatric and Preventive Dentistry, Bharati Vidyapeeth Deemed to be University, Dental College and Hospital, Navi Mumbai 400614, India

About the Authors

Professor Raman Bedi, BDS, MSc, DDS, hon DSc, DHL, FDSRCS (Edin), FDRCS (Eng), FFGDP, hon FDSRCS (Glas), hon FFPH
Emeritus Professor at King's College London.

A former Chief Dental Officer for England from 2002 to 2005, Raman has published over 240 scientific papers, authored 4 books, and examined and lectured in more than 40 countries. He led the team that helped support the passage of three major pieces of legislation: Health and Social Care Act (dental clauses) 2004, Water Act (Fluoridation) 2004, and the Section 60 (2005) order reforming the General Dental Council. In addition he was a member of the Department of Health Top Team and a Founding Member of the National Health and Social Care leadership network.

As Chairman of the Global Child Dental Fund, he has helped support governments around the world to improve child oral health, reaching over 500 million children. He also leads the internationally acclaimed Senior Dental Leadership Programme, a partnership between King's College London, Harvard University, Colgate Palmolive, and Henry Schein.

Andrew Munro, MA, C Psychol, AFBPS
Director at Envisia Learning, heading up its consulting services.

Andrew draws on over 30 years' consulting experience across the corporate, public, and third sectors. Assignments have run the spectrum from graduate recruitment, the validation of selection systems, organisational restructures and redeployment, and implementing career and talent development programmes, through to board-level succession. He has also collaborated on over 150 off-the-shelf and bespoke product applications for individual, team, and organisational diagnostics and tool-kits.

Andrew has collaborated with Raman on a number of leadership development projects and programmes, as well as designing resource material for health practitioners in the area of cultural diversity and inclusion.

He has published in the field of business psychology (*Personnel Review; Selection and Development Review; Executive Development, Assessment and Development Matters*). Andrew is the author of *Practical Succession Management, Now It's About Time*, and *A to Z and Back Again: Adventures and Misadventures in Talent World*.

Mark Keane, MA, PPABP
Principal Practitioner Business Psychologist.

Over the last 20 years Mark has worked in several sectors to produce evidence-based products and programmes.

He is the co-author of *Youth Matters* and creator of the Goliath Index expert system for health and well-being.

Acknowledgements

Our Senior Dental Leadership (SDL) programme has shaped this book as well as the online Advanced Dental Leadership programmes. These have been developed in collaboration with so many people that we are in danger of missing key individuals.

Even so, I want to begin by thanking our academic partners, King's College London and the Harvard School of Dental Medicine, together with our two corporate sponsors, Henry Schein and Colgate Palmolive. This public–private partnership has been very important and has withstood the test of time.

Dr Tom Kennie has been instrumental in developing my thinking on leadership development and I am grateful for our long and enduring friendship. The core SDL team have been great to work with and their role in delivering the programme has been critical, and hence their help with much of the content of this book is acknowledged: Bruce Donoff, Chester Douglass, Jaime Edelson, Jenny Gallagher, Mahesh Verma, Steve Kess, David Lachman, Marsha Butler, and many more who have worked with us over the years.

Aneta Stanev and Noorie Beharry have given the programme the administrative rigour that has been so important and our work would have been more fragmented without their endeavours. The idea of writing the book came from Valerie Wordley and we are grateful for her enthusiasm and perseverance in pushing us to complete the task.

The content of this book has drawn on an array of insights and ideas from our colleagues and programme participants. Several thinkers have also shaped our approach to leadership, in particular those on https://sourcesofinsight.com and the authors of these books:

- *Made to Stick* and *Switch*, Chip Heath and Dan Heath (Crown Business, 2007 and 2010)
- *Mojo*, Marshall Goldsmith (Hachette, 2010)
- *The Manager's Book of Decencies: How Small Gestures Build Great Companies*, Steve Harrison (McGraw Hill, 2007)
- *Help! How to Become Slightly Happier and Get a Bit More Done*, Oliver Burkeman (Canongate, 2011)

Finally, we want to thank all our SDL alumni who over the years have provided so many inspirational stories or projects started and programmes transformed to help improve the oral health of children living in deprived conditions.

Introduction

It is often at the sunset of your career that you reflect on the journey you have undertaken, but when you begin on the path it is just as important to think about where you are going and how to get there. This book is a reflection on one of the most important skills you can learn as a dental professional, but that is not the ability to cut that crown preparation you will learn from your textbooks or now from a YouTube video, or to extract a tooth as effortlessly as you saw performed by your dental school teachers. The key skill to master is leadership to ensure that in your professional journey you start well so that you will finish well.

The competences developed using this book will complement your clinical skills and help you to excel as a dental practitioner. These include interpersonal and communication skills to navigate your engagements with others, as well as personal and professional behaviour, honesty, moral values, ethics, and confidentiality. The book will help you to understand your role and context, evaluate evidence and techniques, make a commitment to self-assessment and peer evaluation, understand maladaptive behaviours and their impact, and maintain your continuing professional development.

The book also outlines actions to take when you encounter incompetence, impairment, or unethical behaviour from colleagues, interacting without discrimination or not being respectful and cooperative. Efficient management of time and resources, understanding the day-to-day running of a general practice, people management, and addressing disciplinary matters to prioritise duties when you face competing demands are covered too. You will discover how to analyse patient safety incidents, and understand the legal and financial contexts of your practice.

Demonstrating effective leadership within your healthcare team to improve safety and quality is an important part of being a dental practitioner. This book will help you serve as a role model for others and demonstrate your competence in an effective manner.

Leadership Skills for Dental Professionals: Begin Well to Finish Well, First Edition.
Raman Bedi, Andrew Munro and Mark Keane.
© 2022 John Wiley & Sons Ltd. Published 2022 by John Wiley & Sons Ltd.

1

Credibility to Make a Good Start

You graduate and obtain a licence to practise and the degree is placed after your name on a business card or plaque outside your surgery. The degree/licence is a sign that you are qualified to practise and that you can be trusted. You are credible. However, credibility is more than a qualification. It is about who you are and how others see you.

> *The most important quality in a leader is that of being acknowledged as such. All leaders whose fitness is questioned are clearly lacking in force.*
>
> Andre Maurois

In this chapter you will learn about:

- The factors that matter in establishing credibility.
- How credibility is based on others' perceptions, requires followers, is better based on actions, is dependent on first impressions, and is fragile.
- Assessing the credibility of your key contacts.
- Auditing what will help or hinder your credibility as a leader.
- Building charisma and distinguishing yourself professionally and commercially.

Overview

Gerald Ratner, former chief executive of the family jewellery company Ratners, achieved notoriety after mocking his own company's products during a speech to the Institute of Directors in 1991. Ratners had built its business on selling cut-price jewellery.

After a liquid lunch, during the speech Ratner stated, 'We also do cut-glass sherry decanters complete with six glasses on a silver-plated tray that your butler can serve you drinks on, all for £4.95. People say: "How can you sell this for such a low price?" I say: "Because it's total crap."' He also claimed the chain gold earrings that were cheaper than a prawn sandwich but probably would not last as long. The Ratners Group lost almost £500 million in value and nearly collapsed.

Credibility is the first hurdle of leadership. If we can't jump this hurdle to project authority and legitimacy, we'll find it difficult to reassure others of our ability to operate

Leadership Skills for Dental Professionals: Begin Well to Finish Well, First Edition.
Raman Bedi, Andrew Munro and Mark Keane.
© 2022 John Wiley & Sons Ltd. Published 2022 by John Wiley & Sons Ltd.

effectively within a leadership role. Skills and competence, no matter how exceptional, will not be enough. Without credibility we will find it next to impossible to succeed as a leader.

What is more, credibility is easily undermined – and once lost it's difficult to regain.

- What factors do you think matter in establishing credibility?
  - Does your credibility depend on a stellar academic track record?
  - Membership of particular networks or clubs, or being an alumni of a certain institution?
  - Experience and age?
  - Interpersonal poise and presentational impact?
  - Or the 'X factor' and charisma?

Think

This section outlines five things to know about credibility.

1.1   It Is Based on Others' Perceptions

One of the hardest tasks of leadership is understanding that you are not what you are, but what you're perceived to be by others.

Edward L. Flom

Credibility is credibility only in the eyes of others. Whatever we might like to think about our talents, contribution, and impact, others are the judge of our credibility. If others don't respect us or see us as credible, we must recognise that perception is a leadership reality.

- Is that unfair? Or is that a reflection of the realities of human nature and social dynamics?

1.2   Our Credibility as Leaders Requires Followers

If we look over our shoulder and no one is following, we're not leading. We can exercise power and status to force others to do what we tell them, although then the result is reluctant subordinates who grudgingly obey our orders, but will not be engaged in our plans. We have credibility when others follow because they want to, not because they have to.

- Think about how your own outlook on credibility will influence the way in which others view you.

1.3   Credibility Is Better Built by Actions Rather Than Words

Dr Rajendra Pachauri is a climate change chief who won a Nobel Prize for coordinating research in climate change, including the warning that the glaciers in the Himalayas might melt by 2035. He came under fire for ignoring his own plea for everyone to reduce their carbon footprint. On the one-mile journey from his home to his office, he could have walked, cycled, used public transport, or the eco-friendly electric car he had been issued. Instead, his personal chauffeur picked him up from his home in a 1.8 L Toyota, ignoring the advice of the Energy and Resources Institute, of which he is Director General, to reduce pollution by avoiding the use of private vehicles where alternatives exist.

As Henry Ford noted: 'You can't build a reputation on what you're going to do. You build a reputation on what you've done.'

We can talk about effectiveness as leaders. We can announce exciting plans for the future and what we intend to do. The reality is, though, that our credibility is established when we deliver against others' expectations.

Don't say it if you don't intend to do it. And if you've said it, do it even if you regret it for being time consuming, awkward, embarrassing, or expensive. If you don't, you will damage your credibility.

This is credibility as commitments and the tough lesson of living with the consequences of misguided commitments should ensure we are more careful when making future commitments.

- What have you done that will reassure others of your leadership credibility?

1.4 First Impressions Count, so Project Well

We only get one chance to make a first impression and that impression is made in a few seconds and is hard to change. People will evaluate us within 10 seconds of meeting us, usually before we've even had a chance to open our mouth.

So be appealing and make sure you get off to a good start in social encounters. Look and sound the part. Beauty is in the eye of the beholder, and others will view you more positively if you establish yourself as credible and confident. To make a positive impact attend to your physical appearance and dress well.

One of the best ways to make a positive first impression is to demonstrate immediately that the other person, not you, is the centre of attention and conversation.

Last impressions matter too. Endings are important. Don't allow conversations and meetings to fizzle out in awkwardness or hesitation. Know how to end social interactions.

- How do you come across to others in social situations?
  - As hesitant and unsure of yourself? Arrogant and more interested in what you have to say?
  - Or as possessing that level of poise and self-assurance that has the confidence to take a genuine interest in others; ask questions and listen; and speak clearly and with power?

1.5 First Impressions: Tactics

- **Prepare in advance** for key encounters, then just try to forget yourself. No one is at their best if they are self-conscious.
- **Be on time** and look the part; present yourself appropriately.

- **Be confident**, and smile; use body language to show you're open to others, make eye contact.
- Avoid a fumbling introduction. Have ready a **'verbal business card'**, a quick, 30-word summary of who you are and what you can do. Focus on the benefits for the other person rather than simply stating your job title: 'I'm X and I'm here to help you with Y.'
- Listen; **remember names** and use them.
- Check your **speaking style**; people judge your intelligence and values on how you select and use words.

1.6   Credibility Is Fragile

Our credibility can be destroyed quickly and sometimes for the most trivial of reasons. The following mistakes will damage credibility:

- **Losing the plot**. When you fail to keep up to date with your field of expertise and fall back on out-of-date thinking and practice, you become out of touch and irrelevant.
- **Questionable ethics**. When the gap between what you say and what you do grows, your credibility disappears into the gap.
- **Being everyone's friend**. Don't aim to be liked, aim to be respected. Attempts to be popular with everyone are seen either as phony and insincere, or as asking for trouble when you need to make tough decisions.
- **Avoiding responsibility**. When you side-step problems or look to blame others, your integrity and leadership courage are rightly questioned.
- **Mismanaging expectations**. Your credibility suffers when you over-promise and under-deliver. Big announcements about future possibilities raise everyone's expectations. And when the reality of results disappoints, your credibility is damaged.

Do

1.7   Assess the Credibility of Your Key Contacts

- Make a list of individuals in a leadership role that you have encountered. Include here colleagues, mentors, your peers, as well as others generally in life you have met who are in some kind of leadership position.
- Rate each on a 1–10 scale of credibility. Don't agonise over your evaluations. It's not a detailed assessment, rather a way of highlighting who you see as more or less credible.
- Review your listing of names and credibility factors (Figure 1.1). Ask:
  - What themes emerge as key factors in those you see as more or less credible?
  - What might this indicate about your own 'theory' of leadership credibility?
  - What might be the implications for what is more or less important to your leadership outlook, and how others perceive your credibility?

Your Contacts	Rating 1-10
Mentor Name	
Peer 1 Name	
Peer 2 Name	
Partner or Family Member Name	
Other Name	

Figure 1.1   Are your contacts credible?

1.8   Conduct a Personal Audit to Ask: What Will Help or Hinder My Personal Credibility as a Future Leader?

Which factors will enhance or undermine your credibility?

- Professional excellence and technical proficiency?
- A track record of outstanding success?
- Your access to influential people and networks, which, by association, boost your own credibility?
- A broad repertoire of leadership capability to get things done effortlessly?
- Exceptional interpersonal and communication skills?
- Charisma to get noticed and to make others feel special?

Be honest in identifying your strengths and any potential shortcomings in order to develop a strategy that ensures you get off to a good start as a credible leader.
What is your key priority? Is it a strength you want to build on – or a gap you know you should fill?

1.9   Build the Charisma Factor

- What will set you apart from your peers and differentiate your practice from others?
  - Is it your professional proficiency?
  - Is it the extent to which you project yourself with authority?
  - Is it how you make others feel special?
- What could you do to project yourself with greater authority, power, and influence?

Review the dynamics of charisma with the help of the further reading at the end of the acknowledgements.

Charisma isn't a magical force. It's the combination of a blend of specific factors: how we project ourselves, how we look and present ourselves, how we listen, and how we interact with others.

- What for you is helping or hindering your personal 'charisma factor'?

In a Nutshell: Credibility to Make a Good Start

To make a good start as a leader you need to establish your credibility. In this chapter you learnt that without followers there is no leadership. Others' perceptions of you are critical.

Also you discovered that credibility is fragile and how to avoid damaging your credibility. How are you perceived by key contacts? What factors affect your credibility? What is needed so you project well and make a good first impression?

In your personal audit, you identified your strengths and potential shortcomings, and put together a robust strategy for personal development.

The chapter finally examined how you can build the charisma factor and understand what will set you apart from your peers.

2

Managing Difficult People

Practical dentistry is as much about handling people as it is about providing clinical care. Not everyone in the dental team or indeed the patients we care for is straightforward. It is important to know the types of difficult people, be aware of how to deal with underperformers and aggression, understand manipulation and flattery, and know which arguments to avoid and how to win those that matter.

> *You only have to do a very few things right in your life so long as you don't do too many things wrong.*
>
> Warren Buffett

> *In order to master compassion, you have to spend time getting to know monsters. When you can do that you will see that there are no monsters, only people that acted like monsters because no one gave them the time or compassion to hear their story.*
>
> Shannon L. Alder

In this chapter you will learn about:

- Recognising some of the different types of difficult people you will encounter, including the tank, the nothing person, and the whiner.
- Dealing with underperformers, including preparation and steps in the conversation.
- Confronting a difficult person, what to do and what not to do.
- Dealing with aggressive encounters, including how to exit the situation.
- Identifying and avoiding others' manipulative behaviour.
- Recognising the motivation behind sarcasm and addressing it.
- Arguments to win and lose, including following the logic of arguments, fighting fair, and defending a weak position.
- Understanding that disagreement doesn't have to be disagreeable, including why the absence of disagreement can be problematic, valuing differences, and remaining on good terms.
- How conflict is inevitable, including avoiding showdowns and listening to be listened to.

Leadership Skills for Dental Professionals: Begin Well to Finish Well, First Edition.
Raman Bedi, Andrew Munro and Mark Keane.
© 2022 John Wiley & Sons Ltd. Published 2022 by John Wiley & Sons Ltd.

- Avoiding questions that you don't want to answer, including redirecting the conversation, keeping it vague, and being direct.
- Appreciating that what people say makes sense to them and may be useful to you.

Overview

They may be in the minority, but 'difficult' people might be the majority reason behind many of the problems we encounter in our professional and personal lives.

It may be a difficult patient who is argumentative or negative, or a difficult colleague who is lazy, or moody, and whose behaviour undermines professional standards. Or even worse, you may have to deal with a substance abuser whose actions threaten the reputation of the workplace.

We are taught at an early stage that teamwork is important in dentistry, but a difficult team member whose tempers and tantrums are disruptive of the clinic dynamic can be a major distraction that affects everyone's work focus.

All too often, difficult people are that way because it has worked for them in the past. They are difficult because their 'difficult' behaviour achieves some kind of pay-off, even if sometimes these pay-offs are counter-productive for the individual in the long term.

This chapter addresses difficult people, difficult behaviour, and the tactics that can be used to minimise their impact on your personal and professional life.

Think

2.1   Difficult People We Encounter

It is a given of life that we will encounter individuals who antagonise, frustrate, annoy, or simply bore us. They're commonly referred to as 'difficult'. Some we simply term irritating, others we call rude, and some we label 'impossible to work or be with'.

There are various ways to deal with different types of difficult people. It probably won't change them, but the tactics you will learn here might help you maintain your emotional equilibrium.

You may encounter various types of difficult people, including the following:

- The **Tank**: confrontational, pointed, and angry, the ultimate in pushy and aggressive behaviour.
- The **Sniper**: rude comments, biting sarcasm, or a well-timed roll of the eyes. Making you look foolish is the Sniper's speciality.
- The **Know-It-All**: seldom in doubt, the Know-It-All has a low tolerance for correction and contradiction. If something goes wrong, however, the Know-It-All will speak with the same authority about who's to blame – you!
- The **Think-They-Know-It-All**: no one can fool all of the people all of the time, but this individual can fool some of the people enough of the time, and enough of the people all of the time – all for the sake of getting some attention.

- The **Grenade**: explodes into unfocused ranting and raving about things that have nothing to do with the present circumstances.
- The **Yes Person**: in an effort to please people and avoid confrontation, says 'yes' without thinking things through. They react to the latest demands on their time by forgetting prior commitments and over-commit until they have no time for themselves. Then they become resentful.
- The **Maybe Person**: procrastinates in the hope that a better choice will present itself. Sadly, with most decisions there comes a point when it's too little, too late, and the decision makes itself.
- The **Nothing Person**: doesn't contribute to the conversation. No verbal feedback, no non-verbal feedback. Nothing.
- The **No Person**: kills momentum and creates friction for you. More deadly to morale than a speeding bullet, more powerful than hope, able to defeat big ideas with a single syllable.
- The **Whiner**: laugh and the world laughs with you; whine and you whine alone. Whiners feel helpless and overwhelmed by an unfair world. Their standard is perfection, and no one and nothing measures up to it. But misery loves company, so they bring their problems to you.

Ask yourself:

- Which of these categories do you encounter the most?
- Which do you find most difficult to deal with?

2.2 Dealing with Underperformers: We Have to Talk

An employee with performance problems is not just your problem, it's a problem for the whole practice team. Other team members will resent taking up the slack for a poor performer. This feeling can permeate the working environment and over time, your excellent performers will vote with their feet, and your service and productivity will suffer.

It's time to talk. This conversation will help do several things:

- **Clear the air**, opening up a dialogue in which issues can be discussed frankly and an action plan agreed.
- **Allow you to** check out your perceptions and assumptions about the individual's performance and the underlying factors to pinpoint specific next steps.
- **Signal to your team** your commitment to excellence and your willingness to challenge any unsatisfactory standards or inappropriate behaviour.

But there are hazards if you mismanage this conversation:

- It becomes an exercise in negotiation in which astute underperformers outmanoeuvre you and you are left feeling powerless to resolve the situation.
- The individual hears what they want to hear, the problem isn't clarified, and no commitments are agreed.
- Emotions – yours and the individual's – run high and the problem escalates into unproductive argument, or, worse, a legal process.

2.2.1 Before the Conversation

What you do and how you think about the issues before the beginning of the conversation will have a huge impact on the outcome. If you spend your time thinking about the other person's bad intentions – real or imagined – and getting outraged, or if you spend your time mulling over the unpleasant things the individual has done or unpleasant conversations you've had with him or her, you're likely to enter the conversation in a negative emotional state and with an antagonistic attitude.

Instead, identify and clarify the problem. Don't jump to conclusions, but do work through in your mind the possible causes and consequences of the underperformance. Just how serious is the issue?

What's your **goal**? What do you hope to achieve from the conversation? If your agenda is to tell the team member off, or show them why they're wrong, you may be setting the scene for a difficult encounter. At this stage it's better to operate to the goal of understanding the individual's perspective and helping them understand yours.

2.2.2 Find a Private Place

No one wants to receive negative feedback in front of others. Sometimes it's unavoidable, but that should be a last resort. Hold the meeting in an office or call the person into a vacant room.

2.2.3 Steps in the Conversation

- **Describe the team member's specific performance issues**. Talk about the issues factually, without mind-reading their motivation or discussing their 'poor effort'. Outline the results of the individual's performance and the impact it is having on others.
- **Describe the expected standards of performance**. Be specific. Don't say they have a 'poor' attitude; instead, list specific occurrences that illustrate problematic behaviour.
- **Reaffirm your faith in the person**. Tell the individual that you still have faith in them as a person and in their abilities; it's their performance level and contribution that need to change.
- **Stop talking**. After you have told the person what specific recent actions were inappropriate and why, stop talking. Give the other person a chance to respond to or refute your statements. **Listen** to what they have to say.
- **Determine the cause of the performance issues**. Does the team member have insufficient training, skills, knowledge? Is there a lack of motivation or incentive? Are there external factors involved (family, financial, etc.)? Are there factors beyond the individual's control affecting their performance?
- **Ask the team member for solutions**. What do they think they could do to improve this situation? Then discuss each solution with the individual. How will it help with the problem? Discuss your own suggested solutions too. Try to jointly improve on and reach the best solution.

- **Define positive steps**. Agree on what future performance is appropriate for the individual. If there are specific things they need to start doing or stop doing, be sure they are clearly identified. If there is something you need to do, perhaps additional training, agree on that as well. Ask the individual to provide their summary. Document the discussion and share the key points and actions.
- **Agree on specific actions to be done and a time frame to implement them**. Arrange for another meeting in the future to track the progress/results of the solution.
- **Schedule in regular review sessions** to discuss progress around clear objectives. Some individuals may decide to leave your work area. Some will rethink their approach and raise their performance; others won't. Work with your human resource professionals to begin a process to exit these individuals whose continued employment can only damage the long-term well-being of your work area.
- **Get over it**. After you have given negative feedback and agreed on a resolution, move on with the job. Don't harbour ill will towards the person because they made a mistake.

2.3   Confronting the Difficult: Dos and Don'ts

If you indicate you will do anything to avoid trouble, that's when you get trouble.

50 Cent

This section gives more general guidance for confronting difficult people in other situations.

2.3.1   The Dos of Confrontation

- **Start quickly and safely**. State the facts: the gap between what you expected and what has happened. Create a 'safe climate' to avoid arousing negative emotions that can only break down a meaningful dialogue. Ensure that you reinforce your respect for the individual by being courteous and polite in the tone of your voice. Check that your body language is communicating respect. And establish a mutual purpose by clarifying your intentions to find a solution that is in everyone's interests.
- **Move things forward.** Look for ways of closing the 'gap'. If you've established the facts, then share your story. Your story is your version of events. It might be wrong, but it is how you think and feel. Use your story to explore the reasons for the gap.
- **End with a question**. Hear the other person's point of view by genuinely listening to discover their story. What do they think happened? Is happening? Will happen in future? Engage others in the problem solving while avoiding any diversionary tactics that fail to address the specifics behind the conflict. Focus on next steps and commitments.

2.3.2   And the Don'ts of Confrontation

- Don't begin the conversation when you are **feeling upset or angry**.
- Don't **'sandwich'** by inserting a tough message within polite pleasantries. You will only confuse the other person.
- Don't **surprise** by suddenly springing an attack on someone out of the blue.
- Don't **play games** with hints and innuendo in the hope the individual will work out how you feel.
- Don't **pass the buck** by blaming someone or something else for the confrontation. The confrontation is between you and the individual. Don't blame anyone or anything else. Take accountability for managing the confrontation.

2.4   Dealing with Aggressive Encounters

> *A Jedi's strength flows from the Force. But beware of the dark side. Anger, fear, aggression; the dark side of the Force are they. Easily they flow, quick to join you in a fight. If once you start down the dark path, forever will it dominate your destiny, consume you it will.*
>
> Yoda

Aggression requires a slightly different approach. You may be on the receiving end of conversations that are:

- **Attacking**: the kind of communication that is threatening and belittling and an attack on you as an individual.
- **Labelling**: a dismissive approach that 'puts you in a box' and defines what you can and can't do through generalisations and stereotypes.
- **Controlling**: a coercive style in which others attempt to dominate and force their views on you (e.g. cutting you off, directive questioning).

You need to see these stratagems for what they are: power games that usually say more about the other person than about you. Don't allow yourself to get caught up in the agenda of someone who is selfish, self-seeking, manipulative, or at times irrational. Instead:

- **Acknowledge the aggression**. Angry people don't want to be ignored. Without encouraging 'bad behaviour', recognise the person's anger. Indicate that you are aware of the intensity of their feelings and are prepared to listen.
- **Stay calm**. Fighting 'fire with fire' is unlikely to be productive, however tempting it may be to respond with your own anger. Maintain your emotional discipline to control any anger you may be feeling about others' unreasonableness. Count to ten. Give yourself the time and space to evaluate the situation, the options, and the implications.
- **Ask questions**. Even the angriest person will eventually slow down once their initial anger has been vented. Ask specific questions – calmly, but not in any patronising way – to discover the issues behind their emotions.

- **Move towards solutions**. Ask for constructive ideas to deal with the situation. Make the other person part of the solution.
- **Be prepared to exit the situation**. After the encounter has ended, don't vent. Repeatedly reviewing, discussing, and reliving the episode will only prolong your negative feelings. Stop yourself any time you catch yourself thinking about what happened.

If someone offers you a gift and you decline to accept it, the other person still owns that gift. The same is true of insults and angry exchanges. In order for there to be any force to the attack, you must first accept it. So decline the 'gift' of aggression.

2.5   Avoiding Others' Manipulative Behaviour

> *The basic tool for the manipulation of reality is the manipulation of words. If you can control the meaning of words, you can control the people who must use the words.*
> Philip K. Dick

Manipulators come in different shapes and sizes. Whatever the tactic – and manipulators draw on a variety of techniques – the aim is the same: to get you to do what they want. Manipulators operate in the following ways:

- Opening up and seeming to talk freely about their own plans, ideas, and feelings. In fact, they're not. Their apparent self-disclosure is calculated to encourage you to reciprocate and provide information that can be used to your disadvantage.
- Beginning the conversation with lots of 'yes' questions to encourage your responsiveness, before shifting to the killer question where they anticipate resistance.
- Using expressions such as 'Don't you think. . .?', 'Don't you feel. . .?' 'Would you agree that. . .?' to push you into what they want.
- Having little hesitation in asking you personal questions at an early stage in your relationship.
- Using emotional blackmail to create feelings of guilt.
- Dramatising and exaggerating to get your attention and sympathy.
- Asking your views about other people and being keen to exchange gossip.
- Looking to force you into making a quick decision about something that is important to them.

If you're aware of these ways of trying to manipulate you, you can more easily recognise them and avoid being taken in.

2.6   Flattery: Nice to Get but Dangerous to Believe

> *Gauge how successful flattery has been by the response it gets: 'Do you really think so?' means they've accepted it; 'Thank you,' means people know they're being flattered; 'Don't talk nonsense' means try again some other time.*
> Guy Browning

Difficult people don't always sound difficult. Sometimes the most difficult people can sound positively charming. And flattery can be one tactic they deploy. Flattery makes us feel good about ourselves. We all want to be liked. We all want to be appreciated. Flattery works, because even we know it's flattery, it's flattering to be flattered.

At best, flattery is a form of sincere compliment. At worst, it is a form of emotional manipulation, creating an expectation of exchange in which the flatterer wants reciprocal praise, or some kind of practical assistance in the future.

The best strategy for dealing with flattery:

- **Accept the flattery with grace**. After all, it might be a sincere compliment. And if it isn't, it's always good to be gracious.
- **Don't get carried away**. Flattery is a variation of Kipling's imposter of triumph: 'If you can meet with Triumph and Disaster/ And treat those two impostors just the same.' See it for what it is: usually an attempt at emotional manipulation rather than praise for your brilliance.
- **Ask yourself what the flatter's motives are**. Without being cynical, think about why you would be the focus of flattery, given the nature of your relationship.
- **Manage any future expectations** on the part of the flatterer. Flattery was their choice; don't let it create any sense of obligation.

> *The trouble with most of us is that we would rather be ruined by praise than saved by criticism.*
>
> Norman Vincent Peale

2.7 Sarcasm

Please, keep talking. I always yawn when I am interested.

2.7.1 Sarcasm as Bad Behaviour

A highly toxic personality in the workplace is thankfully rare. Few patients or colleagues embark on the kind of blatant bad behaviour that is highly disruptive of professional practice. A more common and subtle form of bad behaviour is sarcasm. Though meant humorously and often intended as a joke (and sarcasm isn't always the lowest form of wit), sarcasm is intended to make others look and feel small. It can be extremely hurtful to colleagues and damaging to practice relationships.

What is most important is to recognise the motivation behind the sarcasm, and to be aware of the difference between passive sarcasm (largely humorous and good natured, and a reflection of the individual's general interpersonal style) and aggressive sarcasm that is directed at you personally and intended to put you down.

2.7.2   Choose a Strategy to Address the Sarcasm

There's more than one way to deal with someone who is being sarcastic:

- **Don't acknowledge it**. You can either ignore the sarcastic comment completely, or be 'innocent' of the intention and treat it as a genuine remark.
- **Retaliate** with sarcasm of your own. Here you up the ante and make it clear that this is an exchange where you won't let go and that you will win.
- **Scold**. Point out the sarcasm and the childishness of the person's behaviour.
- **Highlight the motives** of the person. You signal that you are aware of the game that is being played and you are questioning their intentions and what they are attempting to achieve through sarcastic behaviour.
- **Tell them to stop**. If the person's behaviour is consistent, and making you unhappy and having damaging consequences, communicate your feelings directly and request they stop using a sarcastic tone in your interactions.
- **Withdraw**. If the relationship is not that important and the sarcasm is escalating, cut ties completely with the individual.

As with most things in life, context is key in evaluating the best response in any given situation. But if a colleague's sarcasm is beginning to affect your motivation or undermining other relationships at work, find a way to deal with it.

2.8   Arguments to Win and Lose with Difficult People

In a typical argument, each person tries to prove themselves right and the other person wrong. And the outcome is predictable: each person only ends up more entrenched in their views, regardless of who seems to be delivering the dominant argument.

2.8.1   Avoid Arguments You Can't Win

Don't pursue an argument you can't win. Rhetoric and cleverness may win the debating points, but in the process you may make a powerful opponent look foolish and feel humiliated. And they won't forget it. Always give your opponent an escape route they can use with dignity. There are moments of disagreement over fundamental principles when you have to fight your corner and defend your position. There are also many times when the issues don't really matter and you need to let them go.

2.8.2   Remember Your Goal

Marshall your arguments well, but remember your goal. If structured properly, an argument should make a positive case for your viewpoint with supporting evidence, following a clear logic from premises to conclusion. It should also make a negative case against the alternative position to undermine the other's argument.

A different tactic is to realise that arguing will only strengthen the other person's resolve, so the only way to 'win' is to aim for a goal other than being right. The objective is to get the other person to listen and understand your point of view, and to maintain your own inner equilibrium. If you argue with this aim in mind, you may find that arguments become easier and happier.

2.8.3 Fight Fair

Winning an argument is good for the ego in the short term. But it may weaken your character and integrity in the long term. 'Fighting fair' is an explicit understanding of conflict with another party and the willingness to resolve it in a constructive way, as follows:

- **Check your motivation and intention**. Is this an issue worth fighting for? Or am I making a fuss about nothing just to make a point? If it is a big deal, am I prepared to fight fair? Or will I do whatever needs to be done, come hell or high water, to win. . . whatever the consequences?
- **Schedule a time for the 'fight'**. State your expectations in advance to signal your feelings and the issues you are looking to resolve. 'I am feeling upset/disappointed/angry about. . . and we need to work out a way forward. Can we agree a time to discuss this issue?'
- **State the problem**. Don't overdo it by allowing your anger or sense of injustice to exaggerate the scale of the problem and alienate the other person. State the issues objectively, with a clear summary of why you can't allow the current situation to continue. Don't revisit old history and painful memories, but do articulate how you feel now.
- **Don't 'punch below the belt'**. There are rules to the game. Know the limits and keep your arguments within them. There are opinions and accusations you can express that will be so hurtful that you will win the argument, but using them will lose you the game.
- **Ask for change that is fair, practical, and possible**. If you're winning the fight, don't keep pressing to make outrageous demands, designed to reinforce your sense of victory. It will do little to provide a sustainable way forward.
- **Be willing to work out a compromise**. The fight should negotiate changes that work for you and the other party. But don't allow the compromise to end in a vague statement that no one really understands and that each will go on to interpret in their own way. Summarise the agreement and its implications.

2.8.4 Defend a Weak Position

There will be times when you may be 'in the right' but you may also be caught on the hop, ill prepared for a strong opponent who has marshalled a valid attack on your position. You have a number of response options:

- **Stall**: 'Can I come back to you when I have checked the facts?'
- **Dismiss**: 'That point really doesn't seem relevant to the discussion.'
- **Acknowledge but delay**: 'There was a mistake, but right now the cause is unclear.'
- **Escalate**: 'This is a complex issue; I need to talk through the full ramifications with your boss.'

Don't assume that a strong attack from someone else makes you wrong and your opponent right. Before you move to compromise, protect your current position by turning a weakness into a strength.

2.9   Disagreement Does Not Have to Be Disagreeable

If everyone is in complete agreement, either we are charismatic individuals who have persuaded everyone around to our world-view, or we aren't picking up the feedback from others that lets us hear different views. Both are dangerous.

2.9.1   Dangers of Complete Agreement

- **Bland and boring ideas**. Conventional ideas are easily accepted. It is bold and radical ideas that trigger opposition. But as Gandhi said, 'Honest disagreement is often a good sign of progress.'
- **No one cares**. If others are indifferent to an idea, they won't argue. They can't be bothered because they can't see what difference it will make.
- **Others don't understand**. Have you outlined the implications of your plans and what they mean personally to those involved?
- **Others are afraid to challenge you**. Are you exerting too much power and intimidating others? Film producer Samuel Goldwyn was notorious for saying: 'I don't want any yes-men around me. I want everybody to tell me the truth even if it costs them their jobs.' Are you sending out a message of 'my way or the highway'?

2.9.2   Encourage Debate

Purposeful debate, not circular discussion, stimulates a diversity of perspective that generates ideas, spots unusual options, and zeroes in on the best solution. If you're not comfortable debating different views, ask yourself why.

2.9.3   Value Differences

Don't assume that others will always (or should) think like you or that any divergent opinion indicates a fundamental disagreement and the beginning of the breakdown of your relationship. Trust should be about the tolerance of differences. Don't be too quick to put your important relationships in a box – the box of complete harmony – with the expectation that others will always reinforce your beliefs and opinions. They won't and they shouldn't. Others should challenge you. And if they don't, ask yourself why.

2.9.4   Strategies for Disagreeing and Remaining on Good Terms

- **Seek first to understand** and then be understood. Use active listening. If others believe their own point is understood, they will be more receptive to listening to alternative perspectives.

- **Beware of an emotional response**. If you become too emotional your content can be lost in the way you express it. Separate the person from the problem. Stay calm to think clearly about the reasons for the disagreement.
- **Say 'I wonder'**. Rather than introducing your next big idea, begin your conversation with 'I wonder. . .' This signals that you are curious and interested in a specific issue, while at the same time not closing down discussion with others who might begin to second guess your defined views about the solution.
- **Appear reasonable**. Using 'in my opinion' or 'in my experience' (but not in a sarcastic manner) shows that you are not expressing your views as definitive facts and you are still open to debate.
- **Remember your body language.** Your non-verbal communication should match your words. Smile, relax, unfold your arms, keep an open body position, and maintain eye contact.
- **Agree to disagree**. Show support for areas where there is agreement and accept that there will be other areas where there is a divergence of views.

Disagreement is a positive force as long as the discussion remains reasonable, interested, and friendly. You can remain on good terms if you remember it is not always what you say, but how you say it.

2.10 Conflict Management and Achieving Win–Win

The most important trip you may take in life is meeting people halfway.

Henry Boye

There are conflicts to avoid at all costs. There are conflicts to postpone. There are conflicts to face head on – now. And there are conflicts that can be diverted by imaginative thinking and quick decision making. Draw on a combination of imagination and courage to minimise the threat of emerging hazards.

2.10.1 Conflict Is Inevitable

If you aren't experiencing any conflict, ask yourself why. Something is wrong: you aren't pushing hard enough. Don't see conflict as an attack on you as an individual. It is a consequence of the situation you are in and the challenges you're facing. Stand back from any feelings of personal affront. Your personal emotions won't help. Apply your analytical skills to work out the immediate problem you need to overcome to achieve your long-term goals.

2.10.2 Face Up to Conflict Sooner Rather Than Later

If you leave it till later, the issue may escalate into a major crisis. Don't turn every molehill of disagreement into a mountain of brinkmanship. Some issues will go away if you ignore them, but others won't. Keep alert to growing tension and be prepared to respond quickly to defuse the situation. A small gesture or signal can resolve an emerging issue quickly if you are aware of the initial signs of a problem.

2.10.3   Listen to Be Listened To

Sometimes (maybe often) conflict arises because someone else feels their views are not being acknowledged or taken into account. Listening – active listening that hears the real message – is hard work. Improve your listening in these ways:

- Ask questions to summarise and clarify what is being said; don't assume.
- Keep an open mind; don't anticipate what is about to be said and why you disagree.
- Hold yourself back from preparing your next response; don't interrupt.
- Keep your emotions in check to avoid expressing the strength of your feelings; don't let your body language indicate your disapproval.

2.10.4   Avoid Showdowns

Do whatever it takes to avoid this point of conflict. Either you back down (you lose) or the opponent backs down (you still lose in the long run). Never get into a situation when your ego rather than your brain is making the judgement call. Be firm in asserting your demands, but don't allow the conflict to get to the point at which egos are in competition.

2.10.5   Know When to Give In Gracefully

Don't go through life with a battering ram, attempting to break through every obstacle life throws up. Discretion may be the better part of valour. Read the signs to judge when your natural boldness will advance your goals and when it may backfire. Don't keep pursuing a course of action, however courageously, which can only have negative consequences. Ask yourself: is this about me and my pride, or is it a fundamental issue I can influence? If you can't make a difference, retreat.

2.11   Avoiding the Questions You Don't Want to Answer

There are difficult individuals, lacking sensitivity and tact, who seize the conversational agenda through a forthright approach that asks personal questions. Don't allow your good manners to respond openly to inappropriate, intrusive, and intimidating questions. Know who you are dealing with and select the best tactic to manage the situation:

- **Redirect the conversation**, otherwise known as changing the subject! You can seem to build on the question and say 'Now that you mentioned. . .', or just go off on a tangent: 'I am going to get a coffee, do you want one?' etc.
- **Keep it vague**. A generalised response acknowledges the person but provides no content.
- **Smile and say nothing.** This works well in a phone conversation. Don't fill the silence. Wait for the questioner to pick up the conversation.

- **Get distracted.** If in a face-to-face conversation, get up and walk to another part of the room. Look through your paperwork as if you've suddenly remembered something. Take out your phone and check your calls.
- **Repeat the answer you want to give**. Keep a straight face when you repeat your original response, looking directly at the questioner.
- **Be direct**. 'It's a good question but not one I want to answer.' Simply respond politely that you don't want to answer it.

Do

2.12   Difficult People and What They Might Say about You

Eventually we will find (mostly in retrospect, of course) that we can be very grateful to those people who have made life most difficult for us.

Ayya Khema

By any objective standard, some people are just plain difficult. But it's worth asking why we find some specific individuals difficult, and what that tells us about ourselves. It's probably wise to assume that no one ever gets up in the morning and says to themselves, 'I'm going to be difficult today.' What they do makes sense to them. What if that irritating person is as rational, decent, fair-minded, and well-meaning as you are? What could cause them to behave like that?

Difficult people sometimes serve as mirrors we can hold up to ourselves to see what we need to see about our own personality.

In a Nutshell: Managing Difficult People

There is no avoiding the fact that some people are difficult. Who are they? And why are they difficult?

There are some disagreements that can be resolved and others that cannot. Achieving a win–win outcome examines conflict, its inevitability and necessity, and tactics that avoid showdowns.

Constructive conversations provide a structure to prepare and manage some of the encounters with difficult people.

The dos of confrontation highlight starting quickly and safely, moving things on, and ending with a question; and the don'ts emphasise not feeling upset or angry, not sandwiching tough messages, avoiding surprises, not playing games, and not passing the buck.

This chapter asks you to think about the people you find difficult. What might what you've found out say about you?

3

Focus on Your Priorities

Thinking strategically about your clinical development or your career, about what you want to achieve, will provide clarity and focus. Only via active steps to eliminate trivial and unproductive activities will you achieve your dental ambitions.

In the world of 'everything is possible', nothing gets done.

Edric Keighan

In this chapter you will learn about:

- Working backwards to avoid bad strategic moves.
- Prioritising goals by creating urgency for importance.
- Avoiding sunk costs in your personal, professional, and leadership life.
- Uncovering high risk–high reward professional and commercial opportunities.
- Communicating well and obtaining others' commitment.
- Identifying future trends and dynamics with professional and practice implications.
- Mapping out a meaningful, competitive, energising vision.
- Logging your time to improve productivity.

Overview

On 14 December 2004, Don Berwick, CEO of the Institute for Healthcare Improvement, said in a conference presentation to healthcare administrators: 'Here is what I think we should do. I think we should save 100 000 lives. And I think we should do it by June 14, 2006.'

Berwick's Institute for Healthcare Improvement had amassed evidence that the 'defect' rate in healthcare was as high as 1 in 10 and that a high defect rate 'meant tens of thousands of patients were dying every year, unnecessarily'. The Institute proposed six specific interventions that would save lives.

Leadership Skills for Dental Professionals: Begin Well to Finish Well, First Edition.
Raman Bedi, Andrew Munro and Mark Keane.
© 2022 John Wiley & Sons Ltd. Published 2022 by John Wiley & Sons Ltd.

Every hospital of course wants to save lives. But Berwick's path to change was filled with obstacles. First of all, no one wanted to admit that patients were dying needlessly: 'Hospital lawyers were not keen to put this admission on record.' Second, adopting the proposals required hospitals to overcome decades' worth of routines and habits.

Nevertheless, progress was made in signing hospitals up to the campaign. Early adopters shared their successes and supported hospitals that later joined the enterprise.

Eighteen months later, Berwick was able to announce: 'Hospitals enrolled in the 100 000 Lives campaign have collectively prevented an estimated 122 300 avoidable deaths.'

When the destination is crystal clear – 'some' is defined as 100 000 and 'soon' is a particular date – there is a clear direction and focus, and results are able to be achieved.

If Pareto's principle is right – that 80% of our results come from 20% of our efforts – it's useful to think strategically to know where and how to direct those efforts. This challenge addresses the leadership skills of thinking strategically to prioritise time and energy and setting and communicating objectives that coordinate effort.

Think

3.1 Five Things to Think about Concerning Strategy, Planning, and Priorities

3.1.1 Work Backwards to Avoid Indiana Jones's Bad Strategic Move

In the final scene of *Indiana Jones and the Last Crusade*, Jones, his father, and the Nazis arrive at the site of the Holy Grail. Refusing to lead the way to the Grail, the Nazis shoot Indiana's father. Indiana now has to get the healing water of the Holy Grail to save his father. Overcoming several tests, he faces the final challenge: he must choose between scores of chalices, any one of which could be the cup of Christ.

The Nazi leader impatiently selects an elegant golden chalice, drinks the holy water, and promptly dies – the wrong choice!

Indiana chooses a simple wooden chalice, the cup of a carpenter. Unsure that he's made the right selection, he dips the cup into a font and drinks from what he hopes is the cup of life. Discovering he has chosen wisely, he takes the cup back to his father, whose mortal wound the water heals.

This is an exciting scene, but one that highlights bad strategic decision making. Indiana should have given the water to his father without testing it first. If he had chosen correctly, his father would have been saved. But if he had selected the wrong cup, his father would have died, but Indiana himself would have been spared. By testing the cup before he gave it to his father, Indiana had no prospect of a second chance to fight the Nazis. If he had made the wrong choice, he would have died from drinking the water and his father would have died from the wound.

Strategic thinking is the kind that prioritises effort wisely and works backwards, knowing the impact of today's decisions on tomorrow.

- Are you a strategic thinker who sees the long-term consequences of your actions or are you caught up in the pressures of the moment?

3.1.2   First Things First: Create Urgency for Importance

> Set priorities for your goals . . . put first things first. Indeed, the reason most major goals are not achieved is that we spend our time doing second things first.
>
> Stephen Covey

Tasks can be grouped as follows (Figure 3.1):

- Not important and not urgent.
- Not important but urgent.
- Important but not urgent.
- Important and urgent.

Faced with a series of work demands and pressures, it is critical that we know the differences between these categories.

Important and urgent activities are obvious priorities. Unimportant tasks that aren't urgent can largely be ignored. The tasks that jeopardise our overall impact are activities that are important but not urgent. It is attention to these tasks that has the potential to optimise our personal effectiveness. But the lack of urgency means they don't receive the time and effort they deserve.

Manage your competing priorities by creating urgency for long-term important tasks. Keep these tasks on your radar screen, recognising the impact if they are neglected. Do something each day, however small, to build momentum and make progress.

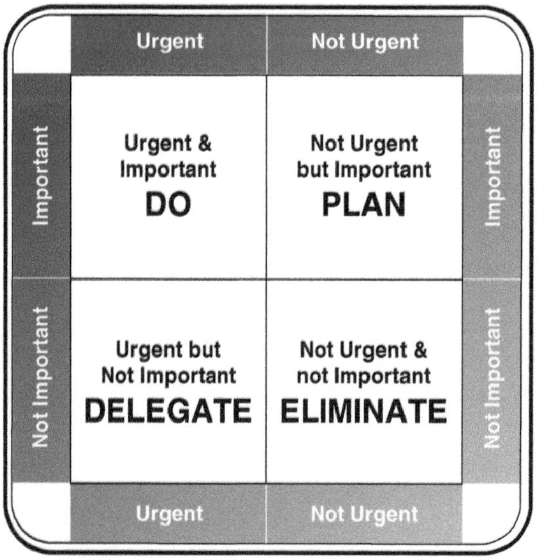

Figure 3.1   Urgency and importance.

- Take a few minutes to reflect on your current commitments to identify those important activities you may be neglecting. These are the activities that will make a big difference to your dental career, but aren't currently registering on your 'urgent' radar screen.

3.1.3   The Law of Sunk Costs

> *Sunk cost: a cost which has been irreversibly incurred or committed prior to a decision point, and which cannot therefore be considered relevant to subsequent decisions.*
> N. Gregory Mankiw, *Principles of Microeconomics*

You pre-order a non-refundable ticket to a sporting event. However, on the night you don't feel like going any longer: you're tired, it's raining, there is a rail strike, and you can watch the event live on TV. You regret the fact that you bought the ticket because you would prefer to stay at home, comfortable on the sofa. But you did buy the ticket. It was expensive and hard to get.

What do you do? If you go to the event, even though you would rather stay at home, you've been caught up in the thinking trap of a 'sunk cost'.

Sunk costs are costs that are irrecoverable. You've spent the money and you won't get it back, regardless of future outcomes. The money is gone, so now you are better off doing what pleases you best. So, unless you can sell the ticket, just forget about what you paid for it. Spend the evening doing what you want to do – watching the game on TV.

The sunk cost factor is played out when we persist in an unproductive course of action ('But I've worked so hard to get to this point'), stick with a bad relationship ('But we grew up together'), or persevere with a project that will never be successful ('But I've invested so much in it, I can't walk away now').

Here are tips to avoid the sunk cost bias:

- Check that you're not sticking with an activity only because of the investment you made in the first place. If it's a bad project (and you can't make it better), get out of it, whatever your initial investment in time, effort, and cost. Cut your losses and move on.
- Allow yourself to make mistakes. Quickly admitting your mistakes is much more productive than persevering with a losing position. Don't worry about 'saving face'; worry about the costs of persisting with an unsatisfactory plan.
- Ask: 'Would I still do it?' Apply the same rigour in examining current activity as you would in planning future commitments. Be prepared to abandon those activities that don't meet the test of 'Would I do it now?'
- Don't confuse your long-term goals with the specific means you've chosen to achieve those goals. Don't stick with an idea that isn't helping progress your goals, however emotionally and financially committed you feel to the concept.

Be honest in your personal audit of the 'sunk costs' in your personal, professional, and leadership life.

- Which activities aren't working for you but you're sticking with because of the past investment you've made, activities that if you abandoned would free up more productive time and energy?

3.1.4   Avoid the Sweet Spot

> *Everybody looks for the sweet spot, that situation in which the risks are low and the rewards are high. The trouble is, that when an obvious situation like that arises, everyone rushes to it.*
>
> B Zeckhauser and A Sandoski

- In the scramble for the sweet spot, 'rewards are diluted and the risks rise'. Look instead at the high risk–high reward opportunities. These might require more time and effort in working through the strategic gains and hazards, but they are the opportunities that others back away from.

It is these possibilities that, with imagination, robust analysis, and shrewd decision making, have the potential to make important breakthroughs. This isn't encouraging reckless expediency, but rather an appeal for bold and imaginative strategic thinking.

- Think strategically about avoiding the 'sweet spot' in your future professional career. Where might the rewards be highest and where will the risks be a potential barrier to your professional peers?

3.1.5   Manage the Dream and Make the Finish Line Nearer

> *Leaders manage the dream. All leaders have the capacity to create a compelling vision, one that takes people to a new place, and then to translate that vision into reality.*
>
> Warren Bennis

Napoleon famously said that 'a leader is a dealer in hope'. This is leadership in the form of outlining a direction for the future that creates the expectation of a better world. It's important then to know how to communicate our thinking and plans and priorities in a way that connects to others – and doesn't confuse or disappoint them.

A good strategy is one that clarifies priorities (what is more or less important) and guides decision making (what we will and won't do). It helps if we communicate our strategy in the following ways:

- **Utilising concrete language**. Employ words about people, activity, and events that mean something practical.
- **Saying the unexpected**. The strategy should make people think and act differently. Outline what it is that makes your strategy distinctive.
- **Telling stories**. If there aren't many examples of our strategy in action, maybe it isn't doing its job too well.

When a carwash company introduced a new loyalty card programme, it tried an experiment. One group of customers received a card that after eight stamps entitled them to a free carwash. The second group got a loyalty card that required ten stamps before the free wash, but they were given a head start. On receiving their card, two stamps had been added. The goal was the same for both customer groups: buy eight car washes and you get one free.

A few months later, the carwash firm evaluated their experiment. Less than a fifth of the eight-stamp customers had come back for a free carwash. Over a third of the head start group had earned a free carwash.

We are motivated when we feel we've made progress. And we find it difficult to motivate ourselves when we have to begin at the very start. When we're kick-starting a project, rather than focus on the novelty of the challenge, it helps to outline the progress that has already been made, and how much work has been achieved to indicate how near we are to the finish line.

- How well do you communicate your plans to others? Do others 'get it' quickly? Or do they seem confused by your priorities?
- Do they feel engaged and energised, or unconvinced and reluctant to commit to your ideas?

Do

3.2 The Future World

> *Most people, out of fear, limit their view of the future to a narrow range – thoughts of tomorrow, a few weeks ahead, perhaps a vague plan for the month to come.*
>
> Robert Greene

It can be difficult to lift our gaze above the moment. But when we do, we find 'the further and deeper we can look into the future, the greater our sense of power' (Robert Greene and 50 Cent, *The 50th Law*). Look ahead for two reasons:

- **Few others do**. If we can think and plan ahead further than others, it provides an important advantage in leadership life. The conviction we project about the future will gain others' attention and command respect.
- **It puts issues into perspective**. If we have a clear view of what matters for the long term and a blueprint of how to get there, we're clear about which issues we can ignore because we know they're irrelevant, and where we need to prioritise our effort.

The following activity works best if you pull together a group of colleagues to share ideas and insights. If that's impractical, you can review it on your own. The aim is to identify a clear set of themes shaping your professional future.

Ask:

- What's not going to change in our field? It's tempting to think 'change is the only constant'. In reality, some things will remain relatively stable. Which are they?
- Which emerging trends (e.g. science, technology) will be key dynamics in changing the face of our field? Why? And what will be the implications for professional and profitable practice?

- Which are the most and least likely scenarios over the next 5 years? In 10 years?
- Which are the areas of greatest opportunity and risk for me personally given my career plans?

3.3   The Vision Test

Google's mission is to organise the world's information and make it universally accessible and useful: a clear, concise, unambiguous, and inspirational statement of intent. What is your vision?

Does your vision:

- Map out a **meaningful** goal, a goal that others connect to and find personally relevant? Will others be committed to this goal, feeling it makes a genuine difference to their lives?
- **Stand out from those of your competitors**? When you articulate your vision, is there a sense of 'wow', this is a bit different?
- **Energise and enthuse others**? Will others feel uplifted and motivated by your plan for the future? Does your vision trigger intense debate about next steps and an urgency to make it happen?

If your proposals aren't connecting to others in a way that is distinctive and energising, you may be failing the vision test. It isn't easy to summarise a clear, distinctive, and compelling vision. It's hard mental work. But it's useful to work through the thought process of asking questions like these:

- What capabilities will make me different as a leader and professional? What specific skills and talents can I deploy as key strengths to help me excel?
- What will make me especially appealing to patients? What factors will help me stand out as distinctive?
- How will I differentiate myself from my 'competitors' and create strategic space to operate profitably?

3.4   Log Your Time to Check Your Productivity

> *Space we can recover, time never.*
>
> Napoleon Bonaparte

Time is your currency. Keep a log of how you allocate your time (Figure 3.2). Review this log at the end of each day and week to identify the productive and unproductive use of your time. Now identify these activities:

- The 'stop dos', time-wasting tasks that are a poor use of your time and not helping advance your goals.
- Those where you could optimise your productivity through greater focus and concentration.
- Those of key importance to your long-term professional well-being that are being neglected or not getting sufficient attention?

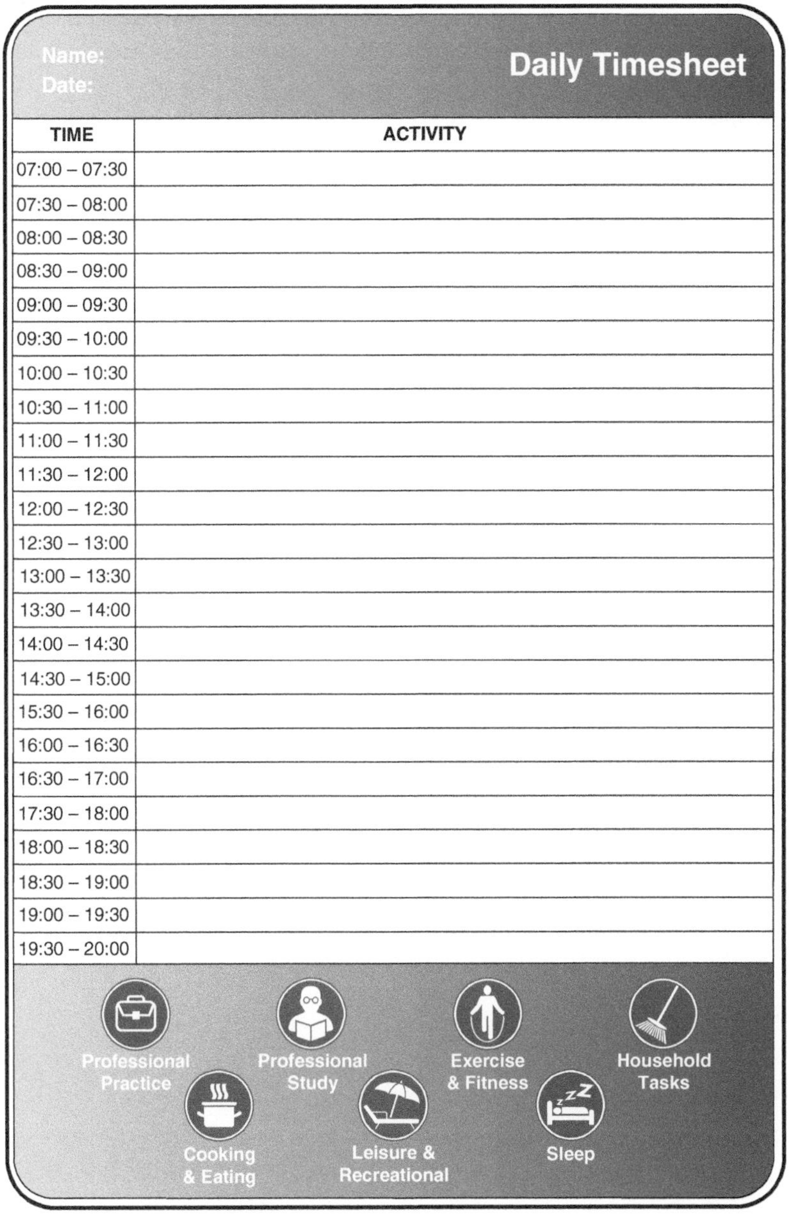

TIME	ACTIVITY
07:00 – 07:30	
07:30 – 08:00	
08:00 – 08:30	
08:30 – 09:00	
09:00 – 09:30	
09:30 – 10:00	
10:00 – 10:30	
10:30 – 11:00	
11:00 – 11:30	
11:30 – 12:00	
12:00 – 12:30	
12:30 – 13:00	
13:00 – 13:30	
13:30 – 14:00	
14:00 – 14:30	
14:30 – 15:00	
15:30 – 16:00	
16:00 – 16:30	
16:30 – 17:00	
17:30 – 18:00	
18:00 – 18:30	
18:30 – 19:00	
19:00 – 19:30	
19:30 – 20:00	

Daily Timesheet

Name:
Date:

Professional Practice · Professional Study · Exercise & Fitness · Household Tasks · Cooking & Eating · Leisure & Recreational · Sleep

Figure 3.2   Taking time to check your time.

In a Nutshell: Direction to Focus Priorities

In this chapter you learnt how to establish your leadership purpose, developed your ability to think strategically, and discovered ways to eliminate trivial and unproductive activities.

The sunk cost bias highlighted those activities that waste your time and energy. You have also found out how to spot high risk–high reward opportunities to advance your career.

Reflecting on how you communicate plans will have enabled you to emerge with a clear set of themes around what is not going to change, emerging trends, likely scenarios, and areas of greatest opportunity.

The vision test has helped you map meaningful goals that engage others. Standing out from crowd, you will be able to articulate your vision with a 'wow' factor.

Remember, in your dental professional life the most important factor that will determine whether or not you achieve your ambitions will be your time – treat it with respect.

4

Values for Leadership Practice

One might say that the business of dental practice is in essence all about ethics and values in your personal leadership. It is therefore important to take active steps to set an agenda for principled leadership in your personal and professional life.

> *You only have to do a very few things right in your life so long as you don't do too many things wrong.*
>
> Warren Buffett

In this chapter you will learn about:

- The significance of values and principles.
- Recognising ethical danger signs.
- Tests to guide ethical choices.
- Managing ego.
- Ethical dilemmas.
- Achieving principled practice.
- Clarifying your own operating principles.
- Developing a personal code of ethics.

Overview

In 1982 McNeil Consumer Products, a subsidiary of Johnson & Johnson, faced a crisis. Seven of its customers had died after taking its Extra Strength Tylenol, capsules that had tragically been laced with cyanide. Within days there was a massive nationwide panic. Initial investigations indicated that someone had tampered with the pill bottles.

Johnson & Johnson faced a dilemma: find the best way to deal with the tampering without destroying the reputation of the company and its most profitable product. From a solid market share of 37 per cent, Tylenol sales dropped to 7 per cent within weeks.

Leadership Skills for Dental Professionals: Begin Well to Finish Well, First Edition.
Raman Bedi, Andrew Munro and Mark Keane.
© 2022 John Wiley & Sons Ltd. Published 2022 by John Wiley & Sons Ltd.

The first step was to alert customers not to consume any type of Tylenol product. As well as stopping the production and advertising of Tylenol, the company recalled all the capsules. Unlike other organisations (e.g. Nestlé and Source Perrier, or Coca-Cola), which downplayed the impact of negative incidents and looked to minimise their accountability, Johnson & Johnson recognised the problem immediately and went public. The second step was to establish and coordinate efforts with the police, FBI, Food and Drug Administration, and media.

James Burke, chairman of Johnson & Johnson, said that, while the poisonings had put everyone in the company into a state of shock, decision making to deal with the problem was in fact simple and straightforward. 'It will take time, it will take money, and it will be very difficult, but we consider it a moral imperative, as well as good business to restore Tylenol to its pre-eminent position,' he said.

Within five months a new tamper-proof Tylenol was on the shelves, and regained 70 per cent of its previous market share.

So how did Johnson & Johnson recover from a precarious position with the potential to destroy its reputation and financial stability? President David Clarke explained the thinking: 'We simply turned to our business philosophy to handle the situation', a credo written in the mid-1940s by his predecessor, Robert Wood Johnson. This credo was a one-page statement of the company's responsibilities to the 'consumers and medical professionals using its products, employees, the communities where its people work and live, and its stakeholders'.

Nevertheless, a reliance on past ethical practice and a 50-year-old credo is not a sufficient set of guiding principles and values for an organisation to continue to operate effectively. In addition, each individual leader has to think about what they believe and why they believe it. We get into leadership trouble when we fail to attend to the values and ethics of professional and business practice.

This isn't about leadership as moralising dogma. Instead, it's about having an internal compass so we know what is important in leadership and ensure that we and others are clear about our principles.

Think

There are six areas to think about in relation to values and principles.

4.1 Words That Indicate There May Be a Problem

- **Just do it**: an invitation to take shortcuts.
- **Make it happen**: cut corners if you have to.
- **I've made my mind up on this one**: a rigid position closed to open debate.
- **Keep me informed here**: nervousness about the decision that's been made.
- **Let's keep the lid on this**: it's an unethical decision, so let's not talk about it.
- **I'm counting on your loyalty**: to keep quiet.

There are also warning signs that may signal unethical practices:

- A gap between formal values and policies and actual practice.
- Subtle pressure to take shortcuts to get things done quickly.

- No or inadequate documentation for important procedures and processes.
- A culture of secrecy.

If you're hearing words that are making you uneasy, you should check for clarification: 'So, what is it you specifically want me to do?'
Ask yourself:

- How attuned am I to the words and actions that indicate integrity (or its absence)?
- Can I read the signs of a working environment based on well-established standards of professionalism, and one that is operating around short-term expediency?

4.2 Four Simple Tests

As leaders we will face genuinely complex moral dilemmas. These are the difficult issues that require deep thinking about the options and their consequences. There are other, easier choices we need to make with honesty about ourselves and our motivations. Here the decision is made against four simple tests:

- **The other shoe**: how would we feel if the shoe were on the other foot?
- **The role model test**: is this a decision we would present to our children as leadership in action?
- **The loved one test**: would we make the same decision if a loved one were on the receiving end?
- **The mother test**: would our mother praise us for this decision?

Ask yourself:

- Which ethical dilemmas have I encountered and had to resolve?
- Was it a genuine 'moral maze' or only a tough judgement because it was difficult personally to do the right thing?

4.3 A Personal Code of Ethics

Legislation and professional codes of conduct provide a framework to define what we should and shouldn't do. But what is your own personal ethical outlook, the beliefs and principles that define you as an individual? It is this set of values that shape your priorities for your professional practice and personal life, the criteria you use in decision making, and the way you deal with colleagues.

Business ethics isn't a form of moral absolutism that arrives at simplistic answers to the range of conflicts and dilemmas we face. After all, it isn't always easy to know what the question is, never mind what the right answer might be. But we do need to understand the complexity and ambiguity of the issues to recognise their significance and develop an informed response.

It's helpful to review different perspectives on ethical decision making. As a starting point, it's useful to ask whether you know what you think about these areas:

- What it means to live the 'good life' and flourish and succeed in your personal and professional life.
- The important professional debates within dentistry.

- The big social issues of our generation: poverty, global warming, crime, diversity, developing-country debt, and so on.

If your response is 'I don't know what I think', it will be useful to invest additional time in formulating your thinking about the following:

- What for me constitutes life and leadership success?
- What are the key issues within my area of academic and professional practice?
- What is my response to today's complex social and political problems?

4.4 Ego: Our Best Friend and Worst Enemy

> *If there's anything more important than my ego around, I want it caught and shot now.*
>
> Zaphod in Douglas Adams's *Hitchhiker's Guide to the Galaxy*

> *The first principle is that you must not fool yourself – and you are the easiest person to fool.*
>
> Richard Feynman

Everyone has an ego. At best, it is our ego that makes us the distinctive person we are. It is our ego that creates our particular persona and projects our unique identity. At worst, it is our ego – selfish and self-seeking – that looks for short-term advantage while operating in ways that are counter-productive in the long run.

We can keep our ego in check in several ways:

- **Staying humble**. It's important to express humility. If others think we 'know it all', they will be less inclined to pass on experience, insights, and ideas that will accelerate our learning.
- **Knowing when to stay quiet and listen**. In the effort to show how clever we are it is easy to dominate conversations. As we do so, we stroke our ego but alienate others.
- **Checking out how others really view us**. A reality check that discovers what others really think about us is tough, but it's key feedback. We should ask those close to us how we are perceived (but avoid reacting badly).
- **Showing, not telling**. If we're good at something, people will see it for themselves – we don't need to tell them.
- **Being generous**. Egotism can lead to selfishness. Altruism gets us further. We should also be generous with our praise of others.
- **Not being hyper-sensitive**. We shouldn't expect everyone to defer to us. Status should be earned and not imposed.
- **Looking at the 'big picture'**. We can keep our ego under control by reminding ourselves of the 'big picture' for long-term success. Short-term wins to boost the ego will undermine more important goals for the future.

Is your ego working positively or negatively for you? At best, your ego helps you advance your goals and stand out as a distinctive professional. At worst, your ego acts as a filter to reality by which you block out important feedback and learning.

4.5 Avoiding the Stupid Stuff

Aspiring US presidential candidate Gary Hart offered a challenge to reporters asking questions about his track record of philandering: 'Follow me around . . . If anybody wants to put a tail on me, go ahead. They'd be very bored.'

One reporter did take up the offer and wasn't bored. Gary was soon discovered with a lovely young woman, and it wasn't his wife. His presidential campaign faltered. Sometimes leaders are the architects of their own downfall.

• Can you identify any risks to your own leadership integrity and credibility?

4.6 Preference Isn't Principle

We should communicate our values and beliefs, the fundamental issues of ethical and professional behaviour. But we shouldn't confuse principles with our own operating preferences – how we as individuals like to work.

Be sensitive to differences and accept that not everyone wants to sign up to your working approach and style.

Do

4.7 Know Why You Believe What You Do

> *To thine own self be true, and it must follow as the day the night, thou canst be false to no man.*
>
> William Shakespeare

Where have your leadership values and principles come from?

• As part of your upbringing and education?
• Working with particular individuals – good, bad, and ugly – who have taught you important life lessons?
• From your own reflections?

Clarify your own operating values:

• Have you worked through your own belief system to know what makes something right and wrong?

If you would feel exposed explaining your leadership values to your peers, take time to work through the issues in your own mind. Could you defend your ethical position in public debate? Don't rely on second-hand opinions. Work through your own belief system to establish the deep-seated principles that are real and authentic for you.

4.8   Key Figures in Your Life

> *Tell me who your heroes are and I'll tell you how you will turn out to be.*
>
> Warren Buffett

Role models can be an important motivational force in our lives. They provide a concrete example of what is possible. Choose the wrong role model, however, and we will end up with a lopsided view of leadership priorities.

Know who in life you admire and why. Don't only look at what they have accomplished, evaluate how they achieved their success.

- List out the three individuals who have had most impact on you in life.
- Why these three?
- What is it that specifically has impressed you?
- How would you describe their values?

4.9   A Principled Practice

First, think about those professions or business activities that have a reputation for operating to high ethical standards.

- What is it that they do or don't do that sets them apart from professions and businesses with a poor reputation?
- How does your profession compare?

Second, ask:

- What constitutes a business or team that is principled, value driven, and ethical? Not in the theory of a 'mission statement' on the wall, but in day-to-day reality?
- How is this practice different to one that lacks clear values and principles?
- How would someone's experience differ between the two?

Third, what are your personal priorities for building and maintaining a principled and value-driven workplace?

In a Nutshell: Values for Leadership Practice

The ethics and values of professional and business practice play an important role in helping you to set an agenda for principled leadership.

In this chapter you learnt how to spot the warning signs of unethical practice, how to push back against any pressure to take shortcuts, and strategies to address moral dilemmas when they arise.

You considered what your personal code of ethics is and how it shapes your personal and professional life and decisions.

Sensitivity to differences is also important, to avoid confusing fundamental principles with personal preferences.

We say in dental professional life that there are two pillars as we look after our patients: Do no harm' and 'Do what is the best for the patient'. This chapter closed by looking at values for your leadership practice and your priorities in building a principled, value-driven workplace.

5

Building and Maintaining Trust

When a patient opens their mouth for you to undertake treatment, there is implicit trust between the two of you. Trust is vital to a successful clinical life and it is important to understand the dynamics of trust, how to build it, and more importantly how to maintain it.

> *Trust is the essence of leadership.*
>
> Colin Powell

In this chapter you will learn about:

- The importance of trust and others' interests.
- Why trust matters and the consequences of its absence.
- The rules of trust.
- The role of daily decencies in building trust.
- Building a trusting environment fostering an exchange of experiences and ideas.
- Valuing difference and embracing challenge.
- Assessing your perception of trust.
- How to forgive.
- Understanding how others receive your behaviour and leadership style.

Overview

On 20 April 2010, an explosion on an oil rig in the Gulf of Mexico caused by a blowout killed 11 crewmen and ignited a fireball visible from 35 miles away.

The resulting fire could not be extinguished and, two days later, *Deepwater Horizon* sank, leaving the well gushing on the sea floor and causing the largest offshore oil spill in US history.

Less than two weeks after the explosion, BP chief executive Tony Hayward told the BBC that while it was 'absolutely responsible' for cleaning up the spill, the company was not to blame for the accident that sank the rig: 'This was not our accident . . . This was not our drilling rig . . . This was Transocean's rig. Their systems. Their people. Their equipment.'

Leadership Skills for Dental Professionals: Begin Well to Finish Well, First Edition.
Raman Bedi, Andrew Munro and Mark Keane.
© 2022 John Wiley & Sons Ltd. Published 2022 by John Wiley & Sons Ltd.

On 25 May, however, BP revealed details of its internal inquiry into the spill and admitted that 'a number of companies are involved, including BP, and it is simply too early – and not up to us – to say who is at fault'.

Hayward made his first and probably most ill-judged gaffe when he told the *Guardian* that 'the Gulf of Mexico is a very big ocean. The amount of volume of oil and dispersant we are putting into it is tiny in relation to the total water volume.'

In an interview with Sky News, Hayward said that the environmental impact of the spill would be 'very, very modest': 'It is impossible to say and we will mount, as part of the aftermath, a very detailed environmental assessment, but everything we can see at the moment suggests that the overall environmental impact will be very, very modest.'

Hayward continued his public relations campaign with a statement to reporters on the Louisiana shore: 'The first thing to say is I'm sorry. We're sorry for the massive disruption it's caused their lives. There's no one who wants this over more than I do. I would like my life back.' The families of the 11 people who died when the *Deepwater Horizon* exploded pointed out that they would like some lives back too.

BP decided to go on the offensive and spent £32m on a national TV advertising campaign in which Hayward pledged: 'For those affected and your families, I'm deeply sorry. We will make this right.' At the same time, the *Financial Times* published an interview with Hayward in which he admitted that BP was unprepared for an oil spill at such a depth: 'We did not have the tools you would want in your toolkit.'

Following a meeting with President Obama at the White House, BP's chairman Carl-Henric Svanberg added to the list of gaffes by telling reporters: 'We care about the small people.'

The full story of the *Deepwater Horizon* disaster is still not known, and no doubt will prove more complex than the media depiction of an exploitative multinational looking to drive down costs through inadequate safety measures. Nevertheless, it is clear that BP's leadership team failed to establish trust: the kind of trust that would have reassured its different stakeholder groups that it was sufficiently concerned to tackle a major disaster.

Trust is a key theme in leadership life. And we run into problems when we think that our professional credibility or technical competence is enough to operate as an effective leader and we neglect the trust factor.

Think

Seven things to know about trust are discussed in this section.

5.1   Trust Is the Trigger of Leadership Reality

Management consultant Peter Drucker said: 'The leaders who work most effectively, it seems to me, never say "I". And that's not because they have trained themselves not to say "I". They don't think "I". They think "we"; they think "team." This is what creates trust, what enables you to get the task done.'

We become a leader when we realise that others' interests are more important than our own and that we can achieve more with and through others rather than by ourselves. This is a recognition that others matter and can make a difference; that we can't do it all by ourselves; and that we can't do it all by command and control.

Is Peter Drucker right? Or is this an overly idealised but impractical view of leadership?

5.2 A Lack of Trust Is Costly

Trust matters and a lack of it can have disastrous consequences.

> *If you don't trust, then what? Many things just don't get done. You're left with doing more and more work yourself.*
>
> D Kouzes and B Posner

Mistrust – being suspicious of others' motivations and dismissing their talents and contribution – makes for a difficult leadership life. As well as the personal cost of long hours and a gruelling schedule, the organisational price is high:

- Under-utilised delegation fails to develop others to take on additional responsibility.
- A lack of team spirit breaks down cooperation and coordination of the overall effort.
- Self-seeking behaviour and political gamesmanship emerge.

The reality is, if we want to be trusted, we have to give some of our power away. And in the process, we gain greater personal power and make a bigger impact.

- Are you an individual who trusts others? Or – deep down – do you feel that most of the time, most people are either lazy or incompetent?

It's worth asking how your attitudes to others will be reflected in your leadership outlook. If you think 'I'm OK but others are not OK', it might be worth revisiting your assumptions about yourself and how you interact with others.

5.3 The Rules of Trust

> *Trust is the essence of leadership.*
>
> Colin Powell

There are some rules that can help you foster and retain trust:

- **Allocate enough time**. Trust needs to be nurtured and maintained. Commit time and effort to keeping in regular touch with others.
- **Don't break confidences**. Don't be tempted to pass on any interesting gossip to others based on a confidence shared by a friend.

- **Don't be too quick to give up** on those who now seem to be 'too much like hard work'. Be patient. Others, like you, will go through difficult passages of life and face challenges that can test any relationship. Be loyal through the tough times.
- **Don't call in too many favours**. Recognise that others have their own priorities. Don't make too many demands on their time.
- **Remember important events** in other people's lives, not simply birthdays or anniversaries, but the key moments that have some particular significance.

5.4   Small Decencies Make a Difference

> *We must not, in trying to think about how we can make a big difference, ignore the small daily differences we can make which, over time, add up to big differences that we often cannot foresee.*
>
> Marian Wright Edelman

Trust is forged in the day-to-day events of life, in the 'small stuff':

- How we acknowledge and greet others.
- The way in which we thank others.
- The emails we send, their content, tone, and timing.
- Remembering the significant times in others' lives.
- Recognising when others are happy or upset.

Trust is built in being alert to the small stuff of 'daily decencies', so we should optimise every opportunity to make a difference.

This is leadership life as courtesy, manners, and grace. And if we struggle to 'be nice to the waiter', we might need to rethink our leadership outlook.

5.5   Trust Creates a Culture of Openness and Honesty

A working environment of trust allows the open exchange of experiences and ideas. This requires:

- A willingness to identify and address recurring problems – not dismiss them as 'one of those things' that happen.
- The motivation to get to grips with the problem – to tackle the fundamental cause, not the symptom.
- A climate that is willing to work through solutions – not to look for reasons why 'nothing ever changes'.

Make it easy for others to highlight problems and failings and admit their mistakes.

5.6 Value Differences

We shouldn't assume that others will always (or should) think like us or that any divergent opinion indicates a fundamental disagreement and the beginning of a breakdown of a relationship.

Trust should be about the tolerance of differences. We shouldn't be too quick to put our important relationships in a box – the box of complete harmony – with the expectation that others will always reinforce our beliefs and opinions. They won't and they shouldn't. Our trusted colleagues should challenge us. And if they don't, ask yourself why.

5.7 But Know Who to Trust and Avoid

If they tell it to you, they'll tell it about you.

Some people will break confidences and share information we have told them that we regard as private.

Some people can't be trusted. They may be:

- **Loose cannons**, individuals with no concept of discretion, who will pass on confidential information to others.
- **Schemers**, who exploit your willingness to share your concerns and worries openly with them.
- **Foolish**, with no insight into good manners and business etiquette.
- **Resentful**, those individuals who are envious of your success and who want to damage you.

Learn to spot these individuals and know how to manage your relationships with them while keeping a personal and professional distance.

Do

5.8 Me and Trust

Make a list of names of people you personally do not trust and then do the following:

- Analyse what it is that makes you distrust them. Is it something specific they've done or their way of doing things generally?
- Did you once trust them but now no longer do? What happened? Are there any common factors? Could one factor be your own behaviour or perceptions?

Reflect on this and ask a trusted friend for their insights on your analysis.

5.9 Forgive

Walking onto the stage for his inaugural acceptance speech, Nelson Mandela shook the hands of the four prison guards who had kept him captive for years. This was a key moment in helping South Africa address its past and move towards a better future.

There is no shortage of 'reasons' for resentment and bitterness. We have all experienced hurt and encountered injustice. But these emotions have great potential for self-destruction. Forgiveness is good and resentment is bad for the soul. Forgiveness, as well as helping you manage the inevitable ups and downs of relationships, improves your own personal well-being.

- Identify an individual you need to forgive in order to be able to let go of any negative feelings and move on.

5.10 The Shoes of Your Clients or Colleagues

Trust requires a level of empathy to see the world not as you see it, but as others experience it, and to 'walk in that person's shoes'.

Put yourself in your clients' or colleagues' shoes.

- Think about the times you have been on the receiving line of leadership. How were you treated?
- Was your trust gained?

Now think how your patients or colleagues may feel about *your* behaviours or leadership style.

In a Nutshell: Building Trust and Maintaining It

This chapter introduced the dynamics of trust, why trust is critical, how to build and maintain it, and the costs of a lack of trust. Valuing differences will steer you away from faulty assumptions about other people. Trust is about the tolerance of differences.

Trust can also be exploited. It is important to know who to trust and who to avoid.

Finally in this chapter, you were encouraged to step into the shoes of your colleagues and patients, and think about how they may respond to your leadership style and impact.

6

Raising Energy Levels

Do you remember that first restoration or dental extraction? I recall being emotionally and physically exhausted and on returning home I went straight to bed. Of course, over time things get easier, but it is important to achieve and sustain high levels of energy to face the challenges of leadership life.

> *Leaders are the stewards of energy. They inspire or demoralise others first by how effectively they manage their own energy, and next by how well they mobilize, focus, invest and renew the collective energy of those they lead.*
>
> J Loehr and T Schwartz

In this chapter you will learn about:

- Managing your personal energy.
- Five life outlooks between short-term satisfaction and long-term meaning and purpose.
- The energy paradox and doing the opposite of crashing out.
- Your comfort zone and getting out of it.
- Keeping something in reserve to meet tough challenges.
- Selling the steak not the sizzle using goal setting and the SCAMPI test.
- Running out of juice and the keys to being revitalised.
- Gaining performance improvement by doing things you don't want to.
- Identifying triggers to raise your energy levels.

Overview

After watching thousands of hours of tennis matches, attempting to identify what the top players did that distinguished them from the others, Jim Loehr found nothing. Then he noticed what players did between points.

The top players had a better way of relaxing after each point in preparation for the next one. During breaks, the less successful players dragged their rackets, muttered under their breath, dropped their head and shoulders, looked around at the crowd distractedly, or even

Leadership Skills for Dental Professionals: Begin Well to Finish Well, First Edition.
Raman Bedi, Andrew Munro and Mark Keane.
© 2022 John Wiley & Sons Ltd. Published 2022 by John Wiley & Sons Ltd.

lost their cool. Giving vent to energy-draining emotions like anger and fear, they looked either demoralised or tense.

The top players, on the other hand, kept their heads high even when they'd lost a point, maintaining a confident posture that telegraphed 'no big deal'. The top players would concentrate their gaze on their racket or touch the strings with their fingers and stroll towards the backcourt, focusing, avoiding distraction, relaxing, and effectively letting the past go. After this mini-meditation, they'd turn back towards the net, bounce on their toes, and visualise playing the next point.

Our leadership effectiveness hinges on the consistency of our performance. And consistency comes from knowing how to re-energise and revitalise ourselves – and others – to prepare for the next set of leadership challenges.

Think

Seven things to know about leadership energy are outlined in this section.

6.1 Managing Our Personal Energy

We can't manage time. However, we can control our energy levels, and it is the way we focus and direct our energy that drives and sustains performance. Bad habits in energy management undermine our productivity; they also constrain our working relationships.

The key to positive energy management – apart from the general principles of a healthy lifestyle – is balancing the expenditure and recovery of energy.

Athletes understand the need to alternate periods of activity with periods of rest.

Over-training – the expenditure of energy without sufficient recovery – leads to burnout and breakdown. Under-training – too much recovery without sufficient demand on energy – results in atrophy and weakness. Energy management establishes an equilibrium between the stress of activity and the renewal of rest.

If the pattern of your life is demanding and intense, ensure that your schedule allows the kind of recovery time that will re-energise you. Rest and renewal aren't best achieved by slumping on the sofa, passively watching whatever is on TV. Choose relaxation and renewal activities that are enriching and absorbing for you, activities that call on a different set of skills. Make time for dancing, yoga, music, sport, whatever it is that takes you out of the pre-occupations of your leadership life and allows you to regroup and re-energise.

- What is your approach to energy management?
- Have you ever thought about your energy levels and how they need to be managed as wisely as your time?

6.2 Surviving or Succeeding: Five Life Outlooks

Marshall Goldsmith suggests that there are five different life outlooks based on the extent to which we derive **short-term satisfaction and happiness** and/or **long-term meaning and purpose** from the activities that command our time and attention (Figure 6.1):

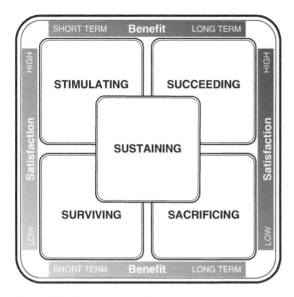

Figure 6.1 Are you succeeding?

1) **Surviving** describes those activities that are low on short-term satisfaction and on long-term benefit. This is the actions in life and work that we have to undertake to keep going and get by. It is a lifestyle driven by chores and drudgery to little end.

2) **Stimulating** identifies those activities that are high on short-term satisfaction but low on long-term benefit. Enjoyable and fun right now (e.g. watching TV, dozing on the sofa), they don't have too much potential to advance our long-term purpose. A lifestyle that is rewarding in the short run, in truth it's in danger of heading nowhere.

3) **Sacrificing** groups together those activities that are low on short-term satisfaction but high on long-term benefit. These are the tasks that we know are important for our future well-being, but not much fun right now (e.g. going for a jog on a dark winter morning, preparing for a tough exam). This is a lifestyle that might be high on the possibilities of future achievement, but without much current joy.

4) **Sustaining** is that cluster of activities with moderate levels of short-term satisfaction that lead to moderate long-term benefits. If not an exactly thrilling lifestyle, it's reasonably interesting and may be life enhancing, with some potential for long-term gain.

5) **Succeeding** defines those activities that are high on both short-term satisfaction and long-term benefit. This is the stuff of life we love doing and, in the process, provides us with great benefit.

It's not a bad exercise to review how we're spending our time in work and outside of work across these five clusters of activity. Everyone has to allocate some time to each. However, if the ratio of surviving to succeeding is looking unfavourable, it's time to check your overall outlook, priorities, and life pattern.

6.3   The Energy Paradox

> *One of the paradoxes of human nature is that the actions that seem most tiring to you when you are at your lowest will raise your energy levels.*
>
> Guy Browning

When you're feeling low, don't make things worse. Don't indulge, crash out in front of the TV, stay indoors, and mope. Instead, do the opposite of what your instincts are telling you to do, however difficult it feels.

Do something you've put off for ages. Tidy the house, embark on a chore you've been avoiding, switch off the TV and listen to a favourite piece of music, go out for a run, call an old friend. Do anything active, productive, and physical. And ignore your body that is saying you're too tired.

6.4   Our Comfort Zone and Getting Out of It

> *We shall have no better conditions in the future if we are satisfied with all those which we have at present.*
>
> Thomas Edison

It's good to focus on personal and professional mastery to build the talents and expertise that move us towards excellence. The downside is that we move into a comfort zone that, pleasant as it is, holds us back from drawing on our full potential and discovering new aspects of our personality. Do you:

- Feel a bit bored and lacklustre?
- Have interesting ideas but don't follow up on them?
- Meet the same people to rerun conversations about the same topics?
- Find yourself repeating the same anecdotes at social events?
- Think you might be missing out on 'something' in life?

If you answered yes, you're probably in a safe and secure phase of your life, but you're also in a zone that isn't stretching and challenging you.

Our comfort zone is that mental boundary within which we maintain a sense of security. When we're out of it, we experience great discomfort. It's also a reflection of our expectations in life now and how we want it to be in future.

Build on your strengths to develop professional excellence, but acknowledge when it's time to get out of your comfort zone.

6.5   Keep Something in Reserve

Deploy effort to fulfil your leadership responsibilities, but don't keep your foot always on the pedal, accelerating at full speed for each and every task you encounter. Don't burn out your leadership engine by over-revving it.

Keep something in reserve for the times when you will need to take on tougher challenges requiring higher levels of energy and persistence.

6.6   Sell the Steak, Not the Sizzle

Leadership is the encouragement of hope for a better future. We shouldn't set expectations we can't meet. Vague dreams and empty promises will disillusion, disappoint, and drain energy levels. Establish goals that meet the SCAMPI test:

- **S**pecific: goals that focus on the detail of what needs to be attained.
- **C**hallenging: goals that require the application of effort around what is possible rather than just reinforcing the status quo.
- **A**pproach: goals that pull us towards positive outcomes rather than push us away from negative outcomes; goals that make us feel good.
- **M**easurable: goals that set a target that can be tracked and evaluated, not objectives with lots of 'wriggle room'.
- **P**roximal: goals with relatively short time horizons, which are more powerful than more distant aims.
- **I**nspirational: goals that we feel are important to us and consistent with our ideals and aspirations for the future.

Talk with passion. Outline an exciting vision of the future. And energise others through your personal enthusiasm. But ground your plans in the realities of the challenges your team faces and in the discipline of robust implementation processes. Sizzle without steak will create disillusionment and resentment.

- Ask the tough question: Do I talk big and act small?

If you sense that you are better at describing your dreams rather than implementing plans to make a difference, it may be useful to shift the balance to thinking smaller and acting bigger.

6.7   Running Out of Juice

Stamina is an underrated attribute for business success.

Richard Moran

- Check your energy levels. Is your own lack of personal enthusiasm having an impact on how you manage your team?
- What might be causing this?
  - Physical or psychological tiredness?
  - Personal circumstances?
  - Your lifestyle?
  - Scepticism and cynicism about corporate life?
  - Other factors? What are these?

Keep your battery charged to stay revitalised. You can't energise others if you're feeling under the weather or under stress.

Do

6.8   Do Something You Don't Want to Do

> *Do something every day that you don't want to do; this is the golden rule for acquiring the habit of doing your duty without pain.*
>
> Mark Twain

- What for you, right now, is a difficult task? This is an activity you know you should do – it will enhance your overall life – but it's proving difficult to find the energy to begin it and complete it. It might be:
  - Waking up and getting up out of bed in the morning.
  - Tidying up your living area to get rid of the clutter.
  - Taking an early morning jog.
  - Contacting an old friend you've lost touch with.
  - Scheduling three hours each week for voluntary activity.
  - Something else.
- Whatever it is, write it down.
- Ask: Why might this task be so difficult for me?
- Now commit to achieving it.
- Treat this activity as an experiment. Note your feelings before beginning the task. And how did completing it make you feel? Less or more energised?

If you're now feeling more positive about yourself, you've gained a new insight: doing what is difficult rather than easy raises our energy.

6.9   Change Your Socks

Odd though it may be, try changing your socks during the day. It's an amazing trick and you will be surprised by how much more energised you feel. Try it.

The aim is to establish a trigger that helps you find a way of reviving your energy level to keep you operating at high performance. Experiment with different tactics, noting what works for you, and build it into your schedule.

In a Nutshell: Raising Your Energy Level

This chapter has explained how leadership effectiveness requires consistency of performance based on optimising energy. Are you surviving, succeeding, or sacrificing short-term satisfaction for long-term meaning and purpose?

You discovered you need to sell the steak, not the sizzle. This emphasises the need to set achievable expectations.

You looked at how to monitor your energy levels to identify whether your own lack of enthusiasm has an impact on the management of your team.

Finally, you undertook an experiment to identify something that will enhance your overall life but that you lack the motivation to tackle right now.

7

Feedback to Keep on Track

A fellow dental student refused to accept any criticism; they saw it as a sign of inadequacy. Not a great characteristic to start one's professional life. We have to understand that feedback is key to our leadership success and it is important to understand how to receive and give it.

> *Ninety percent of the world's woes come from people not knowing themselves, their abilities, their frailties, and even their real virtues.*
>
> Sidney Harris

In this chapter you will learn about:

- Breaking the mirror and accepting feedback from others.
- Pursuing ambitious goals and learning from failure.
- Providing feedback that others value.
- Praising to give others the attention that they're looking for.
- Improving your awareness of excessive praise.
- Knowing who you are working with and how much truth they can handle.
- Improving your awareness of objective feedback, being careful of who you accept feedback from.
- Setting an egg timer to improve your active listening.
- Feeding forward to make progress in the future.
- Evaluating threats to your success by identifying vulnerabilities in your approach that may lead to complacency.

Overview

Trucker Sing Li drove more than 500 miles on a motorway with a cardboard windscreen.

Li refused to replace his van's glass screen after it was shattered by a stone. So he taped thick cardboard to the frame to keep out the wind and then drove by sticking his head out of the driver's window to see where he was going.

Leadership Skills for Dental Professionals: Begin Well to Finish Well, First Edition.
Raman Bedi, Andrew Munro and Mark Keane.
© 2022 John Wiley & Sons Ltd. Published 2022 by John Wiley & Sons Ltd.

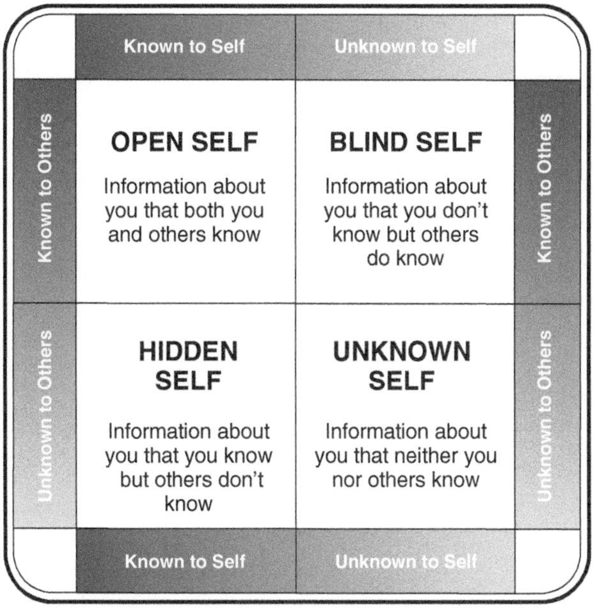

Figure 7.1 Do you know your blind spots?

By the time police arrested him in Henan, eastern China, for dangerous driving, Li's face had turned blue from the cold and one of his eyes was frozen shut.

'I didn't want to fall behind in my delivery schedule and I couldn't afford a repair,' he told a court before losing his licence.

Check your blind spots – those aspects of your behaviour and impact that everyone sees but you don't recognise, which are blocking your view of reality (Figure 7.1). And if you think you're not seeing reality as it is, remove the cardboard from your windscreen.

It's easier, at least in the short run, to keep doing what we've always done. But as leadership coach Marshall Goldsmith notes: 'What got us here won't get us there.' The drivers of our past achievements will not guarantee our future success. Feedback is the reality check to keep us alert to what's holding us back. And we don't get feedback when we put up our 'mental cardboard'.

Feedback is also the leadership skill to provide others with the insight to keep stretching for improvement and gains in performance.

Think

Seven things to know about feedback are explained in this section.

7.1   Break the Mirror

> *Many break the mirror that reminds them of their ugliness.*
>
> Balthasar Gracian

We like to think we are doing well and making an impact. We want to maintain positive feelings about ourselves. Others' feedback can therefore be a difficult experience, providing a reality check that challenges and questions our sense of who we are and what we're achieving. But if feedback is difficult, the alternative – no feedback – is worse.

Without feedback from our work colleagues, friends, and family, we run the risk of continuing to operate in ways that are counter-productive to our interests.

- Make it easy for others to give you the kind of feedback that alerts you to the potential constraints on your long-term success.

7.2 Learning from Failure

The important question is not whether you will fail, but when, and above all, what happens next.

Ed Smith

Don't view every setback as a personal critique of your current effectiveness or a damning indictment of your future potential. Treat failure as a valuable teacher, providing you with learning to refocus your strategy and tactics.

Failure is inevitable if you attempt anything difficult. Directing your efforts to what is easy and trivial won't disappoint, but it won't accomplish anything significant either. Don't let the fear of failure deter you from pursuing ambitious goals. It's far better to fail than to avoid attempting anything worthwhile.

Presentations, conferences, articles, and books showcase success. We all want to hear about what works, discover the reasons, and apply the learning. But these success stories are highly selective.

We should be more open in our discussion of failure – not the kind of failure that is the outcome of incompetent bungling, but the attempts at experimentation that try to do something better but didn't work out.

- Praise failure as an indication of a motivation to make a difference.

7.3 Giving Feedback That Others Value

Feedback is a business term which refers to the joy of criticising other people's work. This is one of the few genuine pleasures of the job, and you should milk it for all it's worth.

Dilbert

How we deliver feedback is as important as how we accept it, because it can be experienced in a very negative way.

To be effective when giving feedback, we must be tuned in, sensitive, and honest. Just as there are positive and negative approaches to accepting feedback, so too are there ineffective and effective ways to give it.

7.3.1 Ineffective Feedback

Ineffective feedback has these characteristics:

- **Attacking**: hard-hitting and aggressive, focusing on the weaknesses of the other person.
- **Indirect**: feedback is vague and the issues are hinted at rather than addressed directly.
- **Insensitive**: there is little concern for the needs of the other person.
- **Disrespectful**: feedback is demeaning, bordering on insulting, or judgmental.
- **Evaluative**: criticising personality rather than performance.
- **General**: aimed at broad issues that cannot be easily defined.
- **Ill timed**: offered too long after the prompting event, or at the worst possible time.
- **Impulsive**: given thoughtlessly, with little regard for the consequences.
- **Selfish**: feedback that meets the giver's needs, rather than the needs of the other person.

7.3.2 How Is as Important as What

You need also to pay attention to how you give feedback. Effective feedback should:

- Be given **promptly**, shortly after the event.
- Contain **encouragement**, emphasising the positive.
- Be **specific**, describing precisely why behaviour is good or not up to standard.
- Be **unambiguous and clear**, not focusing on too many aspects at the same time.
- Focus on **behaviour** and not personal traits.
- Be **individual**, using 'I' statements not 'we' or 'someone thinks'.
- Be **descriptive** rather than evaluative.

Be careful when giving advice as part of feedback. Help the other person to identify the issues and talk through options to build on successes or correct mistakes.

7.4 Praise and Keep Praising

Don't allow any awkwardness or sense of embarrassment hold you back from stating your admiration and respect for others. Criticism, usually indirect, is common. Sincere and positive feedback to provide praise is rare, but much valued.

Most people feel they don't get the recognition they deserve. Ensure that you give your team the attention they're looking for. Notice the small things, the actions or qualities that others are failing to spot, and give full praise for them.

7.5 Excessive Praise

Praise is good for our self-esteem, particularly when we are feeling unsure about ourselves and our capabilities. However, it can have a downside.

Excessive praise is an indication that someone envies us and is setting us up for failure. Or they may be planning to manipulate us to their agenda.

Don't be seduced by flattery. Look for the motive behind it.

7.6   Too Much Truth

A little sincerity is a dangerous thing, and a great deal of it is absolutely fatal.

Oscar Wilde

Truth is powerful, and part of truth's power is in the illumination of reality: seeing things as they are and stating the fundamental issues. Nevertheless, some people may not be ready for this reality, or at least the reality as you present it.

People can find the truth difficult for several reasons:

- It can be **uncomfortable**. We may be extremely unpopular, have bad breath, or be overweight, but we don't enjoy the experience of a colleague pointing out that fact.
- It can be seen as a **challenge**. If you're saying something unpleasant about me, I must think of something unpleasant to tell you. You gave it, so you can take it.
- It can hit a raw nerve and give us a **tough reality check**. We know what the truth is, but we have it hidden away at the back of our mind and don't want to be reminded of it.
- It can be used as a way to deliberately **hurt others**. The other person may fall back on the excuse that they are only telling the truth, but their motives may be far from pure.
- People are used to an **unpalatable truth being sugar coated**, the difficult truth being sandwiched between two positives. White lies have become the social lubricant that we all find acceptable.

Know who you are working with and how much 'truth' they can accommodate.

7.7   Two People Who Tell the Truth

There are only two people who can tell you the truth about yourself: an enemy who has lost his temper and a friend who loves you dearly.

Aristophanes

Be careful who you get feedback from.

Not everyone is able or willing to provide the kind of objective feedback that will support your development. Some may be willing, but don't know you well enough to provide meaningful feedback. And others may know you well enough, but choose to hold back from giving candid feedback in order to protect your feelings.

Do

7.8   Set the Egg Timer

In your conversations, do you wait for others to finish their sentences, standing ready to jump in with your pre-prepared responses? Or do you listen actively, attending to others' views and feelings, and adapt your approach to maintain an authentic dialogue?

Try the egg timer exercise:

- The next time you're in a heated discussion with a colleague, set an egg timer for 60 seconds.
- Let the other person speak for one minute while you listen. The rule is that if you interrupt, the egg timer is restarted.
- Once the other person has finished, reset the timer. Now you spend a minute paraphrasing what the other person has said. Use phrases such as 'I understand you to say. . .', 'I appreciate your views on. . .'
- Only when you have had one minute of paraphrasing are you allowed one minute to comment on the other person's point of view.
- Finally, the other person spends one minute paraphrasing what you have said.

When you're struggling to make headway in a discussion, set the egg timer and you will be surprised by how much progress you make. And in future conversations, debates, and arguments, imagine that the egg timer is on the desk.

7.9 Feedforward Rather Than Feedback

Feedback – giving and receiving it – is an important element of leadership. But feedback focuses on the past and what has happened. Feedforward is about making progress for the future. Feedforward encourages you to ask others for suggestions that will help you become more effective. This is the feedforward process:

- **Pick one behaviour** you would like to change, a behaviour with the potential to make a significant and positive difference to your leadership life.
- **Describe this behaviour** to colleagues you have identified as potential resources for your development.
- **Ask for two suggestions** that might help you make a positive change in the area you have selected.
- **Listen attentively** to the suggestions. Don't comment on, judge, or critique the ideas. Simply listen and thank the person for their insights.
- Then, **review the material** that has been generated to identify those ideas that you want to build on and apply.

In a spirit of humility and learning, try the feedforward exercise and summarise the experience and the outcomes.

7.10 Ten Reasons for Failure

Marc Andreessen, founder of Netscape, the company that lost out to Microsoft in the browser wars of the 1990s, summarised his learning from the experience: 'Keep asking: what are the ten most serious threats to our success? It focuses the mind as much as the prospect of an imminent hanging.'

The answers to the question will focus your leadership thinking on identifying any vulnerabilities in your approach and avoid the hazards of complacency about your current success.

- At your next meeting, congratulate the group on its achievements. Then facilitate a discussion around ten reasons that could lead to failure for you.

In a Nutshell: Feedback to Keep on Track

Without feedback from others, we will not find ways to keep improving as professionals. We also run the risk of operating in counter-productive ways. But receiving feedback can be tough. This chapter has outlined ways to make the process easier.

Giving feedback to colleagues can also be difficult. You have learnt here that how it is given (the process) can be as important as what (the content of the feedback).

You have also discovered that praise emphasises the impact of recognising the small things that others miss, but that excessive praise highlights how to avoid being seduced by flattery.

You are now aware that some of your team may not be ready to accept the truth as you present it, because it may represent a challenge or an unwelcome reality check. You have been encouraged to consider who you are working with and how much 'truth' they can handle.

8

Courage for When It Gets Tough

My nurse once said I was courageous in tackling a difficult extraction of an impacted primary molar. Maybe, but courage is more than undertaking a difficult operation. Courage is evident more in everyday encounters with the people around us. Courage has an impact on our leadership life and on whether fear holds us back from optimising our potential.

> *Promise me you will always remember: You're braver than you believe, and stronger than you seem, and smarter than you think.*
>
> Christopher Robin to Winnie the Pooh

In this chapter you will learn about:

- Leading with challenging goals and time tactics to advance an ambitious agenda.
- Overcoming adversity using the LEAD tactic.
- Allaying anxieties, forging a fearless attitude towards life.
- Building leadership resilience, tackling large adversities by scaling smaller problems first.
- Addressing confrontation effectively and productively.
- Managing conflict conversations using the STATE approach.
- Identifying your fears and how they shape your leadership outlook.
- Using the FASTER tactic and putting your anxious thoughts into perspective.

Overview

On 1 December 1955, Rosa Parks, a 42-year-old African American woman who worked as a seamstress, boarded a bus in Montgomery, Alabama, to go home from work. She was about to initiate a new era in the American quest for freedom and equality.

Rosa sat near the middle of the bus, just behind the 10 seats reserved for whites. Soon all of the seats in the bus were filled. When a white man got on, the driver – following the standard practice of segregation – insisted that all four Black people sitting just behind the white section gave up their seats so that the man could sit there. Rosa quietly refused to give up her seat.

Leadership Skills for Dental Professionals: Begin Well to Finish Well, First Edition.
Raman Bedi, Andrew Munro and Mark Keane.
© 2022 John Wiley & Sons Ltd. Published 2022 by John Wiley & Sons Ltd.

'I did not want to be mistreated; I did not want to be deprived of a seat that I had paid for. It was just time. . .,' she said, 'there was opportunity for me to take a stand to express the way I felt about being treated in that manner.'

She was arrested and convicted of violating the laws on segregation, known as the 'Jim Crow laws'. She appealed her conviction and thus formally challenged the legality of segregation.

At the same time, local civil rights activists initiated a boycott of the Montgomery bus system. It rained on the day of the boycott, but the Black community persevered. Some organised carpools, while others travelled in Black-operated cabs that charged the same fare as the bus, 10 cents. Most of the remainder of the 40 000 Black commuters walked, some as far as 30 km. In the end, the boycott lasted for 381 days. Dozens of public buses stood idle for months, severely damaging the bus transit company's finances, until the law requiring segregation on public buses was lifted.

Rosa Parks's act of defiance became an important symbol of the civil rights movement and an international icon of resistance to racial segregation.

Although widely honoured in later years for her action, Rosa suffered for it at the time. She lost her job at the department store, and her husband Raymond quit his job after his boss forbade him to talk about his wife or the legal case. Both Rosa and Raymond suffered stomach ulcers for years, due probably to the stress of the harassment and fear they had lived in following the bus boycott, and both required hospitalisation. More serious was when Raymond, Rosa's brother Sylvester, and her mother Leona were all diagnosed with cancer within a relatively short period of time, which meant Rosa sometimes had to visit three hospitals in the same day.

On 30 August 1994, Joseph Skipper, an African American drug addict, attacked the 81-year-old Rosa in her home. After his arrest, Skipper said that he had not known he was in Rosa's home but had recognised her after entering. He asked 'Hey, aren't you Rosa Parks?' to which she replied 'Yes'. She handed him $3 when he demanded money, and an additional $50 when he demanded more. Before fleeing, Skipper struck Rosa in the face.

Suffering anxiety on returning to her too small central Detroit house following the ordeal, Rosa moved into Riverfront Towers, a secure high-rise apartment building, where she lived for the rest of her life.

Mark Twain pointed out that courage isn't 'the absence of fear. It is the resistance to and mastery of fear.' And, as the life of Rosa Parks indicates, courage is difficult. But it also inspires the kind of courage from others that can make a big difference.

Think

Five things to know about fear and courage are outlined here.

8.1 To Lead Is to Live Dangerously

> *Exercising leadership can get you into a lot of trouble.*
>
> R Heifetz and M Linsky

Each of us, every day, must decide: do we put ourselves on the line, pushing for what is right and best, or, recognising the challenge and difficulty, get through another day by accepting easy compromises?

Authentic leadership – seeing the long-term gains – chooses the tough and the trouble-some. But wise leadership also judges the timing and tactics to advance an ambitious or controversial agenda.

8.2   To LEAD Is to Overcome Adversity

Before we can lead other people, it helps if we can lead ourselves. And our personal leadership is displayed best not in moments of peace and calm, but in how we respond to the tough stuff of work challenges and uncertainties. Paul Stoltz's LEAD tactic is a useful guide in overcoming adversity:

- **L**isten to our response to adversity. Is our initial response to face the facts and take responsibility, or a groan that life is unfair and we look for someone else to blame or take charge? Developing our facility to listen helps highlight the early signs of adversity and is a reality check on events around us.
- **E**xplore to look at the issues, the possible causes, and evaluate how we see our own personal involvement. Do we see ourselves as utterly at fault and helpless to do anything? Or do we reframe the problem to identify objectively what is and isn't within our control to tackle? Exploration is about perspective, acknowledging where we may have got it wrong and need personally to put things right, while avoiding a disproportionate response where we put ourselves through the mill. In exploration we coolly appraise our ownership of the problem.
- **A**nalyse the evidence is where we begin to evaluate the specifics. This is when we ask the tough questions to assess the scale and scope of the problem. Adversity triggers strong emotions, usually negative, everything from panic to anger to withdrawal and depression. Analysis – grappling with the detail – avoids the thought processes of defeatism, catastrophising, and helplessness. In analysis we stand back to put the adversity into perspective and assess our own resources to respond.
- **D**o is when and how we respond to the adversity. A powerful beginning is to undertake calm reflection about the issues to weigh up the options and identify what we can and can't do. But without action the problem will escalate and we remain stuck. Doing something isn't running around; it's mapping out a sequence of steps that will tackle the situation.

Of course, it's easier said than done to stay rational when adversity next happens. But if we remember LEAD, it may help us put the issues in perspective, identify our own involvement, and realise how we can take ownership to face the challenge.

8.3   The 50th Law: When Fear Isn't in the Driving Seat

> *Fear is a kind of prison that confines us within a limited range of action. The less you fear, the more power you will have.*
>
> Robert Greene

From the beginning of time fear has served a simple purpose: survival. The emotion of fear – triggered in the face of danger – motivated us to flee or defend ourselves. And an awareness of fear meant we could anticipate and avoid future danger.

This power of imagination also had a downside, creating multiple worries and anxieties about potential threats. Instead of being a powerful tactic to cope with danger, fear became a generalised attitude towards life. And as a result we live in fear: fear of expressing ourselves and offending others; fear of disagreement that might trigger conflict; fear of taking the kind of bold actions that drive change but might upset vested interests.

If we can overcome our anxieties, we forge a fearless attitude to life and gain control over our circumstances. Imagine the freedom that results from acting this way:

- Embarking on those actions we would naturally fear.
- Taking the tough decisions we have been avoiding.
- Confronting problems directly rather than playing games.
- Outlining the specific changes we know need to be made rather than accepting unsatisfactory compromises.

8.4   Managing Minor Adversity Well

Adversity spans a spectrum, from the mild disappointment that an exam didn't go well, to the hardship of financial failure, to the awful catastrophe of a safety failure in which lives are lost.

In dealing with maturity with the major adversities of leadership life, it helps if we've experienced and managed the more minor adversities. This is a strategy of building leadership resilience by testing ourselves, climbing the smaller peaks to prepare for the main ascent.

If we lose the plot with the small stuff, we may lack a sense of perspective that responds coolly and calmly to the big stuff.

When we experience small setbacks, it's worth checking our thought processes. Margolis and Stoltz suggest the following prompts:

- **Specific questions** to identify the difference we can make. These are the types of question that ground adversity in practicalities:
  - What aspects of the situation can I personally influence in response?
  - What can I do to make an immediate impact on the situation?
  - What could I do to mitigate the effects of this adverse event?
  - Right now, what do I need to do to make a start?
- **Visualising questions** shift our attention from adversity towards a positive outcome. These questions move us from the current problem to the future solution:
  - What would a person I admire do in this situation?
  - What strengths and resources will I develop in dealing with this event?
  - What will life look like after this adversity has been overcome?

- **Collaborating questions** identify how we can reach out to others for joint problem solving. These questions help us avoid the personal heroics of the lone leader to draw on others' talents and energies:
  - Who else could help me?
  - How can we mobilise the efforts and skills of those who need encouragement or are holding us back?
  - What will see us through this phase of difficulty and hardship as a team?

8.5 The Laws of Confrontation

Not every disagreement or conflict needs to be confronted openly and directly. Some can easily be ignored. But there will be times when leadership courage requires us to be explicit in outlining the issues, explaining why things must change, and negotiating a practical way forward.

8.5.1 The Dos

- **Start quickly and safely**. State the facts: the gap between what you expected and what has happened. Create a 'safe climate' to avoid arousing those negative emotions that can only break down a meaningful dialogue. Ensure that you reinforce your respect for the individual by being courteous and polite in the tone of your voice. Check that your body language is communicating respect. And establish a mutual purpose by clarifying your intentions to find a solution that is in everyone's interests.
- **Move things forward**. Look for ways of closing the 'gap'. If you've established the facts, then share your story. Your story is your version of events. It might be wrong, but it is how you think and feel. Use your story to explore the reasons for the gap.
- **End with a question**. Hear the other person's point of view by listening genuinely to discover their story: 'What do you think happened? Is happening? Will happen in future?' Engage others in problem solving, while avoiding any diversionary tactics that fail to address the specifics behind the conflict. Focus on next steps and commitments.

8.5.2 And the Don'ts

- Don't begin the conversation when you are **feeling upset or angry**.
- Don't **sandwich** by inserting a tough message within polite pleasantries. You will only confuse the other person.
- Don't **surprise** by suddenly springing an attack out of the blue.
- Don't **play games** with hints and innuendo in the hope the individual will work out how you feel.
- Don't **pass the buck** by blaming someone or something else for the confrontation. The confrontation is between you and the individual. Don't blame your boss or organisational policy.

Do

8.6 Manage a Conflict Situation by Having a Difficult Conversation

The ultimate measure of a person is not where they stand in moments of comfort and convenience, but where they stand at times of challenge and controversy.

Martin Luther King

The aim of this activity is not to go looking for trouble and initiate an argument. Instead, the objective is to identify a situation that in one way or another is unsatisfactory and to experiment with a strategy to resolve it. It might be a disagreement with another team member, with a patient, or with a friend or family member.

- Identify the situation and note the key dynamics at work. Then work through the five steps of STATE in preparing for a difficult conversation:
  - **Share your facts.** Keep to the facts. Facts are objective and the least controversial part of your discussion. So get to grips with the details of the facts of the situation and marshal them well to get off to a good start.
  - **Tell your story.** Facts on their own won't advance your position. It is your interpretation of the facts – your story – that is important. Be willing to outline your conclusion, how you interpret and summarise the facts. Ensure that your story is a compelling account and that you keep the facts in perspective.
  - **Ask for others' stories.** You don't know everything and from time to time you will get things wrong. Display genuine humility by asking for others' version of events. Encourage them to base their stories on the facts and how they feel about these facts.
  - **Talk tentatively.** At this stage, expand on your story in the light of others' stories. This is the phase in the discussion where you walk the line between confidence – expressing your facts assertively – and humility – when you are receptive to the reality that you may be wrong. 'Tentative talk' isn't softening the message. It is the recognition of ambiguity and uncertainty to minimise others' defensiveness.
  - **Encourage testing.** Here you are inviting others to open up an authentic dialogue: 'What do you think?' 'What do we need to do to move on?' Some will need encouragement to express opposing views. Others will need your conversational skills to close down ridiculous opinions. But be prepared to review the options before you commit to a final conclusion.

After you have completed this activity, think about the following:

- What was your experience?
- Did STATE work for you?
- What did you learn from the exercise?

8.7   Manage Fear

As we have seen, much of human behaviour is driven by fear. To know fear is to understand ourselves better and be aware of how to provide a response that will reassure and encourage others. The five fears – universal and deep-seated within our natures – are these:

- **Fear of the stranger** and the need for community. We fear those we don't know, and we like those we grew up with and know.
- **Fear of the future** and the need for clarity. The future has uncertainties that create anxieties. We value those who know the future and can provide purpose and direction.
- **Fear of chaos** and the need for authority. We fear disorder and that sense of things being out of control and we need someone to take charge.
- **Fear of insignificance** and the need for respect. We fear that we don't matter, aren't valued, and no one cares about us. We look for the reassurance that we're important and a recognition that our contribution makes a difference.
- **Fear of death** and the need for security. This is a tough one. We worry about what might happen to us, our family, and friends, and we need to feel a sense of security that everything will be OK.

Recognising what you're afraid of and how it shapes your leadership outlook is a tough exercise. It asks you to be honest in the acceptance of fear in your leadership life and to locate the specific fears that might constrain your effectiveness. What are they for you?

8.8   Fear and FASTER

We all experience fear. But when fear is in the driving seat we don't make progress.

- Think of a situation that right now is making you feel anxious and arousing your fear. Now experiment with a tactic called FASTER:
  - **F**eelings. Write down the emotions you're feeling about the situation. Be as specific as you can. If you're feeling unhappy, note the specific feelings you're experiencing about that unhappiness.
  - **A**ctions. Note how this feeling is affecting your behaviour and holding you back from doing what you want to do. Think through the cause–effect relationship by asking: 'So what?' How is this feeling constraining your life progress and outcomes?
  - **S**ituation. What seems to trigger these feelings? What were you doing? Who were you with? What happened or was said that gave rise to the emotions?
  - **T**houghts. Write down the negative thoughts that are running through your head. Note the detail so you can work through the specifics.
  - **E**vidence. At this point, apply the power of rational thinking to interrogate the facts. What would a supportive friend say about the 'evidence' of your thoughts? Are they true – really? Examine the flaws in the logic of your emotions.
  - **R**eview. Revisit your feelings. Look back at the feelings you noted at the beginning of this exercise. Do you still feel as strongly about the feeling? Or have you managed to put the initial emotion into perspective?

- If this exercise worked for you, why do you think that was?
- If it didn't, why not?
- What other tactics might help you manage the negative emotions of fear?

In a Nutshell: Courage for When It Gets Tough

This chapter addressed the importance of courage in leadership, how fear can hold us back, and what to do about it.

Leading to live dangerously asks you to consider the decisions you make each day. Do they produce long-term gains or result in easy compromises?

Through the 50th law – when fear isn't in the driving seat – you examined the role that fear plays in leadership life and the power of being fearless.

The laws of confrontation provided you with a step-by-step approach to outline the issues, explain why things must change, and negotiate a way forward. There are times when you will have to manage conflict by having difficult conversations, and you now know more about how to do that.

9

Influence and Persuasion

With both patients and colleagues, dental professionals are constantly faced with the need to influence those around them effectively.

> *Given the double whammy that people don't think before they speak and that people aren't listening anyway, it's not surprising that communication is our number one problem.*
>
> Guy Browning

In this chapter you will learn about:

- Making others feel special and avoiding superficiality.
- Understanding the realities of human nature, including intentions, the need for reassurance, and bad memories.
- Influencing when not in authority, from knowing what we want, exchange and reciprocity, to sharing credit with others.
- Shifting others' opinions by building on the agendas of trusted individuals and overcoming objections.
- The 90–10 rule of negotiation.
- The science of influence and psychology of persuasion, including reciprocity, social proof, and scarcity.
- Five reasons to keep conversations simple by focusing on the outcomes.
- The nine effective lines of any effective conversation.
- Questions that don't work, including those that require a yes or no response or are intrusive.
- Using charm without overdoing it, including understanding what matters to others.
- Evaluating how 'sticky' your communication is using the principles of SUCCES.
- Using influencing tactics, working through three different scenarios.

Leadership Skills for Dental Professionals: Begin Well to Finish Well, First Edition.
Raman Bedi, Andrew Munro and Mark Keane.
© 2022 John Wiley & Sons Ltd. Published 2022 by John Wiley & Sons Ltd.

Overview

When Jon Stegner saw that his company, a manufacturer, was wasting vast sums of money, he knew he'd have to persuade his bosses to do something.

Stegner asked a summer student to investigate a single item: work gloves. The eager student reported that the factories were purchasing 424 different kinds of gloves, from different suppliers and at different prices. Gloves that cost $5 at one factory were being billed at $17 in another.

Stegner could have summarised the evidence in a single spreadsheet with a single-page proposal for better purchasing cost control. Instead, he collected a specimen of all 424 gloves with their price tags, piled them on the boardroom table, and invited his bosses to see them.

Rational argument based on a well-constructed analysis of the evidence is powerful. Influence that also make things visual and appeals to others' emotions – in Stegner's case 'what a waste' – is even more compelling.

Influence comes in many forms, from the issue of a threat of punishment, through to emotional manipulation and flattery, to persuasive and inspiring presentations. Authentic leadership calls for a repertoire of different tactics for different types of people and situations.

Think

In a world of distracting noise, it can be difficult to get our voice heard. And even if this voice is heard, nothing much might happen. Persuasion and influence are the key skills to ensure that not only are we heard, but when we are heard, things change and we make a positive impact.

This section considers 10 areas to help you think about influence.

9.1   Do You Make Others Feel Special?

Much of the time our working life is conducted at a superficial level. Take the time and put in the effort to make your key contacts – colleagues, patients, and suppliers – feel truly valued. Get to know them, what matters to them, and take a genuine interest in their lives.

It is a willingness to discover the specifics and uniqueness of the individuals you encounter that will make you memorable. Few other people make the effort. If you do, you will stand out.

9.2   Understanding Others: The Realities of Human Nature

> *The master key to human nature is vanity.*
>
> C G L Du Cann, Teach Yourself to Live

Humans come in different shapes and sizes, with distinctive talents and strengths, weaknesses, foibles, and idiosyncrasies, shaped by our varying cultural histories, family backgrounds, life experiences, values, and personalities. However, it is possible to make some generalisations:

- **Most people don't care all that much about you**. As the saying goes, 'Never blame malice for what can easily be explained by conceit.' A lack of caring isn't because most people are mean; it's because they are mostly focused on themselves. You only matter when you matter to someone else. It's not all about you, so don't take it personally.
- **Most intentions are unknown**. We see someone's behaviour and how it affects us, but often we misread the underlying motivation. Don't over-interpret others' behaviours; there may be 101 reasons for their actions. Listen to what they say and get to know them before you jump to conclusions.
- **Selfish altruism explains a lot**. This isn't to say that everyone is selfish and only interested in their own interests. But it is to suggest that you will understand and interact more effectively with others if you recognise the principle of win–win, and how your actions help others and others' actions assume help from you in the future. If you're expecting others to help you simply because of generosity of spirit, you may be disappointed.
- **Bad memories**. Others have a lot of stuff to remember. If they forget you and your priorities, it isn't about you. But do make it easy for others to remember you and your priorities. You are competing for airtime in people's lives with many other voices.
- **Emotions call the shots**. You might conclude a conversation and assume you have had a rational discussion. But most people have stronger feelings about the issues than may be evident from what they say. Because strong emotions aren't usually expressed (from anger at one end of the spectrum to sadness at the other), you won't necessarily know how others feel about you and your proposals. Don't assume that all is well if you haven't recognised the emotional agenda.
- **People need reassurance**. This is out of a mix of confusion about the complexity of life, the need for attention and social approval, and the fear of isolation and loneliness. Others want to feel a sense of belonging and social validation. If you're not making others feel welcome, safe, and secure, you won't connect to them.

9.3   Influencing When You're Not in Authority

You don't have to be a 'person of influence' to be influential. In fact, the most influential people in my life are probably not even aware of the things they've taught me.

Scott Adams

- Think of two colleagues who have or have had the most influence on you. What do they do or say (or not do or say) that increases your willingness to help and support them?
- Now think of two colleagues who have little influence on you. What do they do or not do that reduces your willingness to help?

A formal status may give us a certain leverage in our interactions with others. But because of the interdependencies of different functions, roles, and people, it's probably unwise to rely only on our job title or position with the organisational pecking order to get things done through others. Indeed, resorting to rank may only create resentment.

Our effectiveness and impact will be increased when we develop the interpersonal flexibility to draw on a number of different influencing strategies and tactics. The following are key to influence:

- **Knowing what you want**. If you're not clear about your goals and priorities, you shouldn't expect others to second-guess your intentions and objectives.
- **Being seen as a potential ally**. How do others perceive you? As only interested in others when you want something? Or as responsive to others' requests and generous with your time? It's important to be proactive and to build a base of good will before you need to draw on it.
- **Recognising your allies' world and what is important to them**. Your priorities are not necessarily the priorities of other people. Where do your interests – short and long term – coincide and where might they diverge?
- **Acknowledging the reality of 'exchange' and reciprocity**. This doesn't mean adopting a cynical outlook in interpersonal influence. However, it does highlight an important reality: we have influence insofar as we can give others what they need in exchange for what we need. Exchange is conducted through many different currencies (e.g. emotional acceptance, information, contacts, practical assistance). Know what others want and what you can give them.
- **Sharing credit with others**. It's difficult to be brilliant alone. Our efforts are typically the outcome of cooperation and collaboration. The more credit you share, the more you will motivate others to work with you, and share the benefits of future activity.

9.4 Shift Others' Opinions

> *Power and influence are not the organisation's last dirty secret but the secret of success for both individuals and their organisations.*
>
> J Pfeffer

It is difficult to make our voices heard in the 'communication clamour', however personally engaging and charming we are.

To make more of an impact, it helps to understand the fundamentals:

- **Focus your influence on the key opinion formers**. You don't need to get your message across to everyone.
- **Link your position to a credible individual or source**. Don't advance an 'out-of-the-blue' proposition. Build on the arguments of trusted individuals.
- **Anticipate the objections others will raise and deal with them**. Recognise likely resistance in advance and know how to overcome opposition.
- **Don't appear to be one-sided**. Draw on qualifiers and counter-arguments to establish yourself as a moderate and mature individual.
- **Be direct**. State your conclusion clearly to leave others in no doubt of your proposals or recommendations.

- **Encourage others to join in and make the argument their own**. Don't assume that your views will be accepted instantly. Work through the issues to allow others to make them real and personal to them.
- **Use repetition to reinforce your message**. Don't over-elaborate and go off at a tangent.
- **Make your argument simple and easy to comprehend**. End with a clear conclusion and recommendation and a commitment to action.

9.5 The 90–10 Rule of Negotiation

> *If you spend all your time arguing with people who are nuts, you will be exhausted and the nuts will still be nuts.*
>
> Scott Adams

For any negotiation, 90% of the result is determined in the first 10% of the negotiating time. The other 90% of the time is needed to settle the last 10% of the details. And the first 90% is determined by three factors:

- Do you like the other party?
- Does the other party like you?
- Do you like the idea?

If the answer is no to one or two out of the three, don't waste time on pointless discussion – the negotiation will never result in a satisfactory outcome.

9.6 The Science of Influence and the Psychology of Persuasion

> *It is much more profitable for salespeople to present the expensive item first, not only because to fail to do so will lose the influence of the contrast principle; to fail to do so will also cause the principle to work actively against them. Presenting an inexpensive product first and following it with an expensive one will cause the expensive item to seem even more costly as a result.*
>
> Robert B Cialdini

When Robert Cialdini was researching the science of influence, he decided to go beyond the typical academic review of the research literature. He went undercover, taking on a variety of roles where persuasion and influence are key to success, working in car sales, fundraising, and telemarketing. From the combination of his research and summary of practitioner practice, he outlined six principles:

1) **Reciprocity**. Think of this as 'You scratch my back; I'll scratch yours'. If you do something positive for someone, they'll do something good for you. If you do someone a favour, they tend to feel indebted to you and want to pay you back somehow.
2) **Commitment and consistency**. When people are presented with an idea or appeal that fits their self-image, they are very likely to accept that idea. This is the phenomenon

of consistency. And people who make commitments tend to follow through with those commitments. They have decided, through consistency, that a certain action coheres with who they believe themselves to be.

3) **Social proof.** 'Monkey see, monkey do.' This is the idea that people will do what other people around them are doing. You see a group of people looking up into the sky. What are you going to do? You're going to look up into the sky too.

4) **Authority**. Most people will respect authority figures who have an important message, an effective style, and a platform from which to speak.

5) **Liking**. The people most likely to be influenced by you are people who like you. Physical attractiveness also plays its part here.

6) **Scarcity**. If people think that something is going to run out, they will rush to buy it.

9.7   Five Reasons to Keep Conversations Simple

Some conversations twist and turn in different directions and spiral into complex debates. Enjoyable as a late-night activity with friends, these conversations rarely result in a meaningful outcome in the workplace. And there are other conversations that make a difference, concluding with clear outcomes. These are the conversations to keep simple, for these reasons:

- **Clarity avoids misunderstandings.** The more you say, the greater the scope for different meanings to be taken from your words. Simplicity based on brevity provides a clear message.
- **Emotional power**. Your emotional message and tone are lost in the muddle of many words. Express the intensity of your meaning through fewer words.
- **Avoid boredom**. Short and simple communication holds others' attention. Unnecessary and irrelevant details make for dull conversation.
- **Keep your ego at bay**. Elaborate arguments within a complex conversation might demonstrate your education and intelligence. They might also be a barrier to listening to and understanding others' perspectives, and to engaging others in the key issues.
- **Focus**. When you want to conclude with a commitment to next steps, a short and simple conversation works best.

Know the kind of conversation you should be having. And if it's a conversation that should end in a clear outcome, keep it simple.

9.8   The Nine Opening Lines of any Effective Conversation

There are only three 'story lines' for triggering a conversation:

- Something about the **situation**
- Something about the other **person**
- Or something about **you**

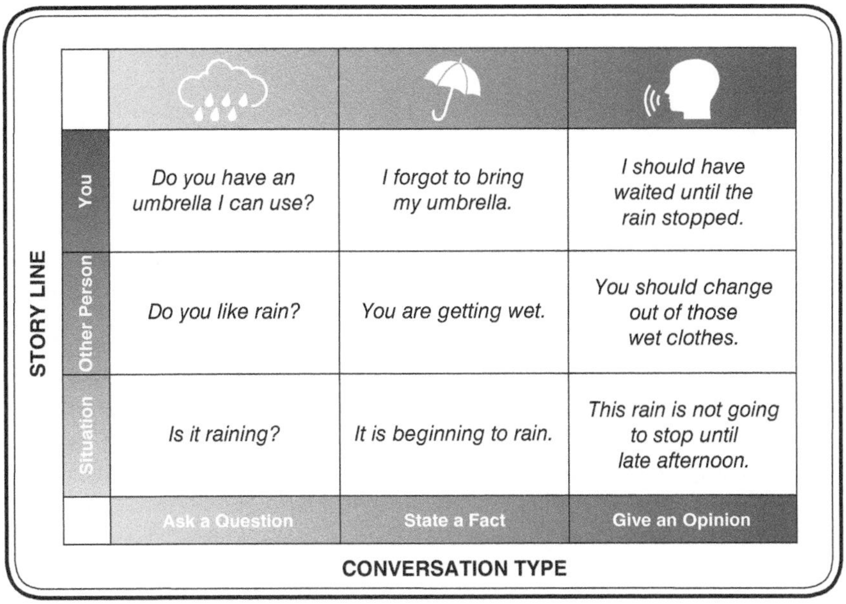

STORY LINE — You	Do you have an umbrella I can use?	I forgot to bring my umbrella.	I should have waited until the rain stopped.
Other Person	Do you like rain?	You are getting wet.	You should change out of those wet clothes.
Situation	Is it raining?	It is beginning to rain.	This rain is not going to stop until late afternoon.
	Ask a Question	State a Fact	Give an Opinion

CONVERSATION TYPE

Figure 9.1 Conversation starters.

And there are only three ways to initiate a conversation:

- Ask a **question**
- State a **fact**
- Or give an **opinion**

That gives nine permutations of ways to trigger a meaningful conversation (Figure 9.1).

The most effective strategy, if you're not completely sure of yourself, is to comment on the situation you and the other person are in. It's low risk and makes it easy to evaluate the other person's interest. But if you're feeling more confident, then ask the other person about themselves, although do it in a way that opens up the discussion.

9.9 Questions That Don't Work

There are some sorts of questions that don't work:

- Those that **generate a 'yes or no' response** and can kill a conversation if the other person isn't in the mood to keep the discussion going, e.g. 'Are you feeling OK?'
- Those that are **intrusive** and an invasion of others' privacy, e.g. 'So why aren't you married?'
- Those that are **threatening** to others and make them back off, e.g. 'Why the **** did you do that?'
- Those that **indicate you are superior** and others are inferior, e.g. 'Why do I have to do everything myself?'
- Those that **require guesswork**, e.g. 'Do you know why I think this department is no longer fit for purpose?'

Know why you're asking a question:

- Is it to engage and involve others in a meaningful conversation?
- Or is the question designed to put up a barrier to block authentic communication?

9.10 Using Charm Without Overdoing It

Charm is getting the answer yes before you've even asked the question.

Albert Camus

Benjamin Disraeli, a flamboyant dandy and writer of romantic novels, did not seem to be the kind of individual who would become a pillar of the political establishment in Victorian England. His maiden speech in the House of Commons in 1837 was poorly received. After enduring a great deal of jeering and barracking, he ended with the words, 'Though I sit down now, the time will come when you will hear me.'

By 1874, he had become a favourite of the Queen, leader of the Conservative party, and, after his defeat of his long-standing adversary William Gladstone, prime minister of the United Kingdom. Quite some political recovery.

One princess remarked, 'When I left the dining room after sitting next to Mr Gladstone, I thought he was the cleverest man in England. But after sitting next to Mr Disraeli, I thought I was the cleverest woman in England.' Disraeli understood the power of charm.

Charm is a powerful force, one with the potential to engage those sympathetic to our beliefs, to persuade the undecided, and to overturn opposition from our adversaries. However, charm can be overplayed to the point that its strength becomes a weakness.

Here are some ways to be charming:

- **Don't be boring**. We are prepared, albeit reluctantly, to acknowledge some personal shortcomings. We will happily admit to a bad memory or poor timekeeping. But we won't accept that we are boring. Being boring is one of the new deadly sins of modern life.
- **Get to know what matters to others and notice the little things**. Make others feel special. Much of the time life is conducted at a superficial level. Take the time and put in the effort to make others feel truly valued. Get to know them, what matters to them, and take a genuine interest in their lives. It is a willingness to discover the specifics and uniqueness of the individuals you encounter that will make you memorable. Few other people make the effort. If you do, you will stand out. And spot those things about individuals that others often take for granted and don't appreciate. The big stuff is obvious (e.g. awards or certificates on the wall, family or holiday photographs, interior décor, clothes). Charm others by noticing the little things that they find important, but others miss. Recognise the personal details and draw attention to them. It will make others feel good about themselves and, in turn, positive about you and your contribution.

- **Never tell it the way it is**. Your assessment of 'it' may be wrong and one that isn't shared by anyone else. In addition, you may be locking yourself into an indefensible position that undermines your credibility. No one wants to hear 'it' as it is. They want to hear 'it' in a way that makes them feel positive about themselves.

Do

9.11 How 'Sticky' Is Your Communication?

John F Kennedy outlined his goal: 'put a man on the moon in a decade'. This is a powerful idea, with the key elements of a 'sticky' idea that people understand and remember, and that changes the way they think and behave. Check that your communication meets the criteria of stickiness by following the principles of SUCCES:

- **S**implicity: a single clear mission.
- **U**nexpected: put a man on the moon.
- **C**oncrete: a clear definition of success.
- **C**redible: from a powerful source, the US president.
- **E**motional: with appeal to the aspirations and instincts of an entire nation.
- **S**tory: how an astronaut has to overcome great obstacles to achieve an amazing goal.

9.12 Analyse Martin Luther King's 'I Have a Dream' Speech

There are few more well-known or powerful speeches than that given by civil rights leader Martin Luther King, Jr, on the steps of the Lincoln Memorial in Washington, DC., on 28 August 1963.

- Watch the video clip of Martin Luther King's speech at https://www.youtube.com/watch?v=3vDWWy4CMhE.

The most famous paragraph, embedded in the middle of the speech, is as follows:

I have a dream that one day this nation will rise up and live out the true meaning of its creed: 'We hold these truths to be self-evident: that all men are created equal.' I have a dream that one day on the red hills of Georgia the sons of former slaves and the sons of former slave-owners will be able to sit down together at a table of brotherhood. I have a dream that one day even the state of Mississippi, a desert state, sweltering with the heat of injustice and oppression, will be transformed into an oasis of freedom and justice. I have a dream that my four children will one day live in a nation where they will not be judged by the colour of their skin but by the content of their character. I have a dream today.

- Why do you think this speech was so influential?
- Look at some of the analysis of the speech that is readily available online to identify how and why the words had so much influence.

9.13 Influencing Tactics

Read through the following scenarios. For each of the three scenarios, take two to three minutes to do this exercise:

- **Analyse the situation** and the factors that might be at work. What might be going on that you are not aware of? What assumptions might you be making or others making about you? How might you be perceived?
- **Note what you might do subsequently**. What next steps might be relevant? What might you have learnt about yourself?

1) You are part of a project helping out children in your local community. Feeling rather pleased with yourself and your commitment to voluntary activity, you are shocked to discover that the children are laughing at you, your appearance, dress sense, and accent.
2) You are invited to lead a project team to identify opportunities for local students to collaborate on voluntary projects in the developing world. After several hours of unproductive discussion and a lack of creative thinking, it is clear that the six members of the group are finding it difficult to work together.
3) You join an established work team in a new job. At the end of the first week, you are surprised when one of the senior leaders asks to speak with you. It is clear from the conversation that your language has offended one of the team and he has indicated he found several of your jokes offensive.

Review your thinking about each scenario:

- What dynamics might be at work?
- How easy or difficult was it to identify with each of the three scenarios?
- What might you now do to establish influence and make a positive impact in your own leadership role?

In a Nutshell: Influence and Persuasion

This chapter has looked at why you need influence as a leader and how to be effective. What influence do you have with colleagues, patients, and suppliers? Do you make them feel special, know what matters to them, and take a genuine interest in their lives?

Discussion of the 'communication clamour' highlighted that it can be difficult to make your voice heard. How can you gain attention and shape others' opinions? The ongoing conversations you have with patients and colleagues matter. The nine effective story lines of conversation provided you with a framework for different types of encounters.

Thinking about questions that don't work encouraged you to think about the purpose of your questions and their effectiveness.

Your analysis of Martin Luther King's 'I have a dream' speech will have illustrated how words matter for influence.

This chapter also helped you review the dynamics of your relationship with someone who you need to understand but don't.

10

Working with Teams

Dentistry is a team business. So you should yourself ask how effective you are in team management so that both you and those around you can have a more productive and fulfilling leadership life.

> *When team members regard each other with mutual respect, differences are utilized and are considered strengths rather than weaknesses. The role of the leader is to foster mutual respect and build a complementary team where each strength is made productive and each weakness irrelevant.*
>
> Stephen Covey

In this chapter you will learn about:

- The signs of effective teams, why they succeed and fail.
- Rules of teamwork in setting operational ground rules.
- Avoiding the role of team problem solver.
- Coordinating the distinctive talents of the group.
- Breaking free from the preservation of harmony to encourage critical thinking.
- Working with diverse teams, including clarifying behaviours, standards, and expectations.
- Managing team conflict, harnessing productive conflict, and addressing destructive behaviour.
- Turnaround strategies for underperforming teams to identify and resolve problems.
- Building an extended team, including those in other work units and elsewhere.
- Your own team style and how to approach teamworking.
- How teams develop: forming, storming, norming, and performing.
- Building a team for life, identifying where you need to prioritise and focus and where you are spending time that is counter-productive.

Overview

IBM – Big Blue – was in trouble. Set for the biggest loss in US corporate history in 1993, it was seen as a 'dinosaur, implosion, and wreck', and was planning a major break-up of its operations to ensure its survival.

Leadership Skills for Dental Professionals: Begin Well to Finish Well, First Edition.
Raman Bedi, Andrew Munro and Mark Keane.
© 2022 John Wiley & Sons Ltd. Published 2022 by John Wiley & Sons Ltd.

Outsider Lou Gerstner was brought in to oversee the corporation's anticipated gradual decline. On arriving at HQ, Gerstner noticed signs saying 'Team' all over the offices. He asked: 'How do people get paid?' The answer: 'We pay people based on individual performance.' Gerstner's initial analysis was of an organisation driven by politics and turf wars, in which the cooperation and collaboration of teamwork were non-existent.

Gerstner began a programme to implement a transformational strategy to keep the company together, refocus on the IT services business, embrace the internet, and revive its culture. His starting points were:

- Open up channels of communication throughout IBM.
- Attack the elitism within the senior management population to disband the bureaucracy of committees and bring together people who 'can help solve the problem, regardless of position'.
- Fire the political players who preferred games to reward those people who were team players.
- Focus on the customer. In 1993, IBM's customers 'felt betrayed and angry about its pricing and lack of responsiveness'. Gerstner announced that the organisation would now put the customer first, with the message that it was there to serve its clients.

The combination of teamwork and a focus on the customer isn't in the book of 'innovative breakthrough strategies', but it's an operating philosophy that seems to work.

When we move away from 'I know best and take it or leave it', we shift to a successful business model that draws on the collective talents and energies of others to respond to changing patient requirements.

Think

Nine things to know about teamwork are explained here.

10.1   Teamwork: Why Teams Succeed and Fail

> *It is amazing what can be accomplished when nobody cares about who gets the credit.*
> Robert Yates

Teams fail when:

- Trust breaks down and team members lack respect for each other's contribution or are suspicious of others' motives.
- Interaction is ineffective and unproductive; some members talk too much, others' contribution is overlooked, and discussion fails to generate practical outcomes.
- There is a lack of role clarity or clear understanding of individual and team accountabilities.
- In the absence of an energising purpose and specific goals to clarify team outcomes and success.
- There is a lack of discipline around information flows, meetings, and follow-up.

And the signs of effective teams are:

- The willingness to talk to each other with candour, rather than behind one another's backs.
- A respect for differences of view and the encouragement of intense debate.
- The maturity to deal with conflict, and to know when it doesn't matter and when it needs to be escalated into a frank exchange.
- Care and concern for each other and the willingness to provide intellectual and emotional support.
- A recognition that more can be achieved through team coordination than through the sheer brilliance of any one individual.

Be a team player. Accept that you can't pursue your personal agenda without a full consideration for the views of others. Be prepared to compromise and agree solutions that work for your colleagues, not just for you and your own goals.

10.2   Teamwork: The Rules

Teams work more productively if they know the rules of engagement. These are the values and principles that clarify the scope of the team; the nature of its interactions, norms, and expectations of support and challenge; how it manages disagreement and conflict; and the nuts and bolts of team discipline and manners. Take time to clarify the team's ground rules and everyone's expectations of how it should operate before you get going.

10.3   Avoiding the Role of Team Problem Solver

Never tell people how to do things. Tell them what needs doing and they will surprise you with their ingenuity.

Theodore Roosevelt

We should make our experience and expertise available to our colleagues. But we shouldn't become the focus of others' problems. Keep pushing problems back for others to resolve. Ask searching questions and provide insights to facilitate their thought processes – but don't solve all their problems. Here are some tips:

- **Hand the problem back**. Don't solve the problems that others present. Pass the problem back, but do it with prompts and questions to help others find the solution. And be clear about expectations – your expectations of them, and your role in helping them deal with the problem.
- **Ask for a written summary**. This isn't to add to life's paper shuffle. It is asking for the discipline of clear thinking that a written analysis can provide. It helps translate vague

thoughts into a clear understanding of the situation, the issues, and working through the pros and cons of different options.

- **Connect others to a supportive colleague**. It's tough to grapple with a new and unfamiliar problem on your own. Make connections to those who can help access expertise, knowledge, and skill to solve the problem.
- **Involve others in implementation**. It's not much fun to do the hard work of problem solving to see others get the credit for implementing the solution. When you delegate work, allow others to see progress from start to finish and take ownership of the full problem-solving process.

10.4   The Sum of Its Parts

Is the whole greater than the sum of its parts?

A good team isn't just a collection of individuals who work together. An excellent team is the result of the interaction of individuals, drawing on the full range of distinctive skills within the group.

- Are you playing your part to coordinate these different talents through shrewd work allocation and delegation?
- And do team members have a good understanding of each other's talents?

If not, conduct an exercise in team awareness to ensure there is a clear understanding of the diversity of its capability.

10.5   The Groupthink of Teamwork

'How could we have been so stupid?' demanded US President John F. Kennedy after his administration's bungled invasion of Cuba.

Worried about Soviet plans to move into the US's 'backyard', the Kennedy administration embarked on an attempt to overthrow the Castro regime. The result: a humiliating defeat at the Bay of Pigs.

Was it stupidity? No: the operation's planners included some of the smartest people in America at the time. The administration failed because it allowed groupthink to mismanage the forces of disagreement, debate, and conflict in planning the mission. It was groupthink, not stupidity, that was the dynamic behind the Bay of Pigs fiasco.

Groupthink is the phenomenon that arises when teams work together but there is a need to preserve harmony, no one wants to be the voice of dissent, and critical thinking is subordinate to a position of power.

If everyone is in 'agreement' with your views, you're in leadership trouble.

- Encourage debate and challenge within your team to ensure that different views are heard and worked through.

10.6   Working in Diverse Teams

The choice is not diversity or homogeneity; the choice is between well managed diversity and badly managed diversity.

David Crawford

Do diverse teams perform better than work groups that are more homogeneous? Yes and no is the answer. To analyse the reasons is to identify what we need to do to harness the gains of diversity for greater productivity and innovation.

Diversity is a double-edged sword. As Sarah Louise Muhr observes, 'the diversity literature is vast in both the disadvantages and advantages of diversity'. In the short run, diversity can be difficult. It just seems easier to work with those who are like us and who like us. And homogeneous teams get on better and feel more comfortable working together. The price of homogeneity may, however, be failing to sustain team effectiveness over the long run. Over time, homogeneity seems to create the kind of cognitive complacency and interpersonal lethargy in which performance levels fall.

Diversity keeps us on our team toes. The variation of different team member perceptions, opinions, and ideas keeps the work group fresh and challenged, introducing that constructive conflict that triggers creativity. It also helps avoid the hazard of groupthink in which team members suspend their critical thinking in favour of group consensus.

But team diversity also has the potential for miscommunication, team member anxiety, and conflicting goals.

As Scott Page suggests, rather than asking 'Why can't we all get along together?', it may be better to ask the practical question 'How can we be more productive together?' and understand the key processes of problem solving, conflict management, and creativity. If we're not proactive in how we approach these activities, then we shouldn't be surprised when diversity becomes a barrier and blockage to effective teamwork.

In working with diverse teams:

- **Expect different expectations**, but be prepared to discuss them openly. This is partly setting standards and ground rules, but also checking each individual's expectations: of you and the level of support they require from you, the team, the task and criteria for success, their own role, others within the team, and what is reasonable and fair.
- **Establish relationships of trust**. Without trust, others won't feel able to discuss the real issues that concern them. Trust isn't engendered overnight; it takes time to create an environment in which communication is genuine and conflict is managed constructively.
- **Clarify team standards and behaviours**. Here it can be helpful to draw up a team contract, an agreed set of rules to guide interaction that is respectful and considerate. The team contract should also outline the consequences of breaching the agreement.
- **Encourage team members to share** their different experiences, knowledge, and ideas. These differences are the assets that enhance task problem solving and creative thinking, but are often neglected. Use team-building exercises to improve the flow of communication and keep your team energised.

- **Apply a policy of zero tolerance** to discrimination and any behaviour that is disruptive and disrespectful. This isn't a strategy of teamwork through lectures about employment policy. It is about building an atmosphere in which individuals are respected as individuals, and team members feel confident in challenging bad behaviour.

10.7 Managing Team Conflict

Where all think alike, no one thinks very much.

Walter Lippmann

When we bring together people from different backgrounds with varying aspirations, experiences, and abilities to work together, conflict is inevitable. Conflict can be constructive: it creates a dialogue in which ideas battle and the competitive process fosters creativity. At worst, though, conflict within the work group is a destructive force that fosters resentment, holds back innovation, and delays decision making.

When creative conflict looks like it is spiralling into destructive behaviour, your options are these:

- The **direct approach**: confronting the issue head-on to solve the problem and impose a solution.
- **Bargaining**: helping others find a compromise through give and take.
- **Enforcement** of team rules: reminding a difficult team member of the ground rules for teamwork and outlining the implications of disruptive behaviour.
- **De-emphasis**: highlighting the areas of agreement and downplaying the extent of the disagreement and conflict.

Different tactics can be deployed at different times, depending on the nature of the conflict, the maturity of the team, and your own preferred leadership style. But destructive conflict can't be avoided.

10.8 Turnaround Strategies

If you've taken over an underperforming team, resist the urge to fire-fight and do something immediately. Instead, take time to form your own views by finding out the facts and talking to everyone who interacts with the team, internally and externally. Use your judgement and experience to identify the cause of the problem. Do any of the following descriptions fit this team?

- **Lethargic**: a team without enthusiasm, drive, or motivation.
- **Incompetent**: a team with low levels of expertise and big gaps in knowledge.
- **Confused**: a team with little understanding of the organisation's goals and unsure of their specific roles.
- **Inefficient**: a disorganised team with poor time management and little coordination and cooperation.

- **Unproductive**: a team with low output, a poor understanding of commercial realities, and weak decision-making skills.
- **Badly behaved**: a team characterised by rivalry, gossiping, back-biting, and conflict.

Once you're clear about the issues, put in place a response that addresses the underlying causes. To turn around an underperforming team:

- **Identify how the team got that way**. Ask the tough questions, speak to the right people, but don't jump to conclusions. Analyse all the information you can get before making your diagnosis.
- **Gain an insight into team members' strengths and weaknesses**. Recognise the different contributions that are made based on hard data, not just on what someone tells you.
- **Resist fire-fighting**. Knee-jerk reactions won't help. Turnaround strategies aren't quick fixes, they're about rebuilding a team that will continue to perform well in the long term.
- **Where you can, pick your team**. Some members may stay, some may go. Plug the gaps in knowledge, experience, creativity, etc. Identify those individuals who are supportive and able lieutenants.
- **Start the process of rebuilding the team's reputation**. Look for early wins that can help change perceptions and also build morale.
- **Set out challenging but achievable goals and expectations**. Ensure they are understood by the team and build in regular monitoring. Clarify lines of accountability.

Turnaround strategies can take time. As the team regains credibility, draw on this to raise its profile and access additional resources to make progress.

10.9   Build an Extended Team

> *If you build a network, you will have a bridge to wherever you want to go.*
>
> Harvey Mackay

Direct your attention on the immediate practice team to ensure it is performing effectively. But don't overlook the 'wider team' in which you operate: your peers in other work units. And access the knowledge, expertise, and skills of individuals outside the practice, individuals with the potential to become your extended team.

Develop your networking skills and contacts to build new relationships. Networking is often associated with a focus on 'Who can I meet who can help me advance my goals?' This is the kind of networker who attends conferences to swap business cards with other delegates. Most of the time, this is a waste of time.

Network with an attitude of 'Who can I help?' This shift in emphasis will build the kind of relationships that will make you part of a bigger team.

Do

10.10   Your Team Style

Have you thought about what type of role you typically take on in a team? When is this role more or less helpful? Does your preferred role always 'work' or do you need to be flexible in taking on different roles?

- Select a team (academic, sports, or other) of which you are either a member or which you lead.
- Now assess your approach to teamworking – which of the below fits you best?
  For each of these, consider how flexible or versatile you are in taking on this role. Is this something you find comfortable or do you struggle?
  - Encourager
  - Compromiser
  - Leader
  - Summariser/clarifier
  - Ideas person
  - Evaluator
  - Recorder
- Having reflected on the variety of roles and contributions that lead to effective teamwork, what are your priorities for your own development?
- Which aspects of teamwork do you want to explore more?
- Which types of roles will you look to take on?

10.11   How a Team Develops

One of the most widely used explanations of how a team develops was provided by Bruce Tuckman, who explains four stages:

- **Forming** – the leader gives guidance and direction, roles are typically unclear, and there are questions around the team's purpose, objectives, and relationships.
- **Storming** – team members jostle for position, there may be challenges, there is an increase in understanding of the team's purpose, but still some uncertainty, sub-teams and cliques may form, and the team needs to focus on goals to avoid these distractions.
- **Norming** – the team reaches consensus and roles are understood, decisions are made by the group or delegated to individuals, the team starts to enjoy the sense of community, processes and working style are discussed, and the leader is respected.
- **Performing** – the team has a shared vision and can get on with achieving its goals, disagreements are resolved positively and necessary changes are made, team members look after each other, and the leader delegates and oversees, but does not need to instruct or assist the team.

Using an example of a team you were in that developed from scratch, how did the following happen?

- What did you do at the start of the team?
- How did you get to know each other?

- How did you explore the diversity of people in the team, their strengths, preferences, and habits?
- What did you do in times of difficulty or crisis?
- How effective was the team in fulfilling its purpose?

How well does Tuckman's model reflect how the team developed?

10.12   Build a Team for Life

Review your current set of personal, social, and professional contacts. Write down the names of your current team members. This group is the beginnings of your extended team.
Now work through this list:

- Where, right now, within your **current set of relationships**, do you need to prioritise and focus additional effort?
- Where should you be forging those relationships that will work for the long term?
- Who are you spending time with that is **potentially counter-productive** and will not help you advance your longer-term goals?
- Who on the list has the contacts to connect you and open up new networks to keep extending your team?

This isn't an exercise in ruthlessly culling friendships. It is, however, an activity to identify who now or in the future will become your extended team, and the relationships that will or won't help you advance your goals.

In a Nutshell: Working with Teams

Why do some teams succeed and others fail? This chapter set out the 'rules' of teamwork, and the values and principles that clarify the scope of a team, including how disagreement is approached.

As a team leader, you have examined how you draw on the varied talents within your work group.

You now know that team conflict can be constructive or destructive. What makes the difference?

Turnaround strategies identify the reasons why a team is underperforming, and how to address the underlying causes. Do you have the confidence to build an extended team, including peers and those in your wider network, to access their knowledge, expertise, and skills?

11

Change to Implement Excellence

Every student reflecting on their future clinical life aspires to provide excellent dental care. However, the day-to-day routines all too often constrain that aspiration. The solution: maintaining that passion for excellence will require a change in lifestyle.

> *Where does leadership begin? Where change begins.*
>
> James McGregor Burns

In this chapter you will learn about:

- How moments of relaxation can improve performance.
- Fostering a culture and climate that encourage innovation.
- Managing change, including using ADKAR.
- The language of change 20-60-20 and typical responses to it.
- Finding the bright spots that are worth replicating.
- Thoughts and feelings – the Rider and the Elephant.
- Assessing how good is good and moving ahead of complacency.
- Developing a T-shaped mind to catalyse excellence.
- Moving from the current situation to the future desired state with energising word pairs.

Overview

Change requires creativity. And in the analysis of what makes creative people creative, an intriguing fact emerges. Creative individuals make a life choice to be creative. It's true that creative people are curious and open-minded, and comfortable with ambiguity and uncertainty. But a key factor is the decision to make creativity part of their personal identity.

Brasil Tata is a Brazilian manufacturer of steel cans. It's not at first examination a very imaginative business, but it's a company that has one of the best reputations for innovation in Latin America.

Brasil Tata pioneered innovation when new employees were asked to sign an 'innovation contract'. There is the expectation that every new employee will be a future inventor to

Leadership Skills for Dental Professionals: Begin Well to Finish Well, First Edition.
Raman Bedi, Andrew Munro and Mark Keane.
© 2022 John Wiley & Sons Ltd. Published 2022 by John Wiley & Sons Ltd.

stimulate organisational creativity, and that individuals will bring their ingenuity and innovation into the workplace.

The company also simplified processes to make it easy for employees to submit their ideas. In 2001, when a severe energy crisis forced Brazil's government to give businesses a strict quota of electricity, Brasil Tata's employees dreamt up hundreds of power-saving ideas. Within a few weeks, the company's energy consumption had fallen by 35 per cent, reducing it to below quota, so the company could resell the extra energy. In 2008, employees submitted 134 846 ideas, an average of 145 ideas per individual.

- How do you define yourself? As someone looking to get by? Or as a creative and innovative pioneer striving for excellence?
- And how do your colleagues see themselves? As actively engaged in innovation to keep pushing for improvements?
- How do you engage your colleagues in the process of creative change?

Think

Six things to know about innovation and change are outlined here.

11.1 Thinking like Leonardo da Vinci

> *The greatest geniuses sometimes accomplish more when they work less.*
>
> Leonardo da Vinci

Michael Gelb has been asking the question 'Where are you when you get your best ideas?' of thousands of people over the years. The most common answers include 'in the shower', 'resting in bed', 'walking in nature', and 'listening to music'. Almost no one, Gelb observes, claims to get their best ideas at work.

Writing about Leonardo da Vinci, Gelb notes that the artist took regular breaks from his work. Even when working on the masterpiece *The Last Supper*, he spent several hours in the middle of the day lost in daydreams. Ignoring the exasperation of his employer, who wanted him to work more steadily, Da Vinci responded, 'It is a very good plan every now and then to go away and have a little relaxation. When you come back to the work your judgement will be surer.'

Sometimes creative thinking does involve the hard work of research and thinking. Sometimes it also requires us to take a break and allow the rhythm of our subconscious to do part of the work for us.

11.2 The Soil of Innovation

> *Rather than telling the plants to grow, we need to tend to the soil in which they can.*

How creative are those you work with? Creativity isn't simply about the presence of a few highly original thinkers and innovative problem solvers, important though these individuals are. Look at the culture and climate of your work area to determine if it encourages or discourages innovation.

- Does your team feel motivated?
- Is your team challenged and keen to explore new possibilities?
- How much fun is there in your work area?
- Does your team have freedom to think and authority to apply new solutions?
- How much time do team members have to stop and think?
- Are you providing support to those who question and challenge?
- What level of trust exists within the team?

Introduce creativity techniques to stimulate imagination and innovation. But also look at the 'soil' in which your plants are expected to be creative.

11.3   Where Change Starts

Change is not only likely, it's inevitable.

Barbara Sher

The issue is not whether change will or won't happen. The issue is whether we manage the process proactively or allow events to overwhelm us. Start change in your own work area by thinking ADKAR:

- **A**wareness of the need for change: is your work area happy with the status quo, or is there a sense that improvements need to and can be made?
- **D**esire to participate and support the change: are you on your own, or is there a real enthusiasm from your team that looks to make a contribution?
- **K**nowledge of how to change: what level of insight and understanding exists within your team about the realities of introducing and implementing change?
- **A**bility to implement the required change: what capability can you draw on? Do you have specialist expertise and technical know-how, as well as skills in project management, communication, and political influence?
- **R**einforcement to sustain the change: after the initial enthusiasm to make improvements, what infrastructure is in place to follow through to make things stick?

Look to introduce ideas that make improvements within your work area. But go into the process with 'your eyes wide open' by analysing the energy, purpose, skills, and talents within your team to contribute to your change management enterprise.

11.4   The Language of Change: 20-60-20

Whenever we introduce a change we can generally predict that around 20% of the people will jump on board, no matter what it is. Another 60% kind of hang back, playing the game of wait and see. The remaining 20% reject the change out of hand, regardless of what it can offer.

CEO, from Paul Stolz, *Adversity Quotient*

If you are introducing change, you should listen to the vocabulary of those around you:

- Great. We should have done this years ago. When do we get started? This is the sound of the enthusiastic 20 per cent.
- How will this affect me? Will my job stay the same? What will be the impact on the team? This is the language of the 'wait and see' 60 per cent.
- We tried this years ago. Here we go again. Change for change's sake. Impossible. This is the noise of the rejecting 20 per cent.

Of course, the language of change isn't always matched by behaviour and actions; some individuals are good at making the right noises in briefings and meetings, but they behave very differently afterwards.

However, it's useful to listen to the words people are using, and how loudly they're saying them. And if your best people are making negative noises, maybe you should rethink your strategy for change.

11.5   Begin with the Bright Spots

Faced with a scenario of dismal results, an underperforming practice, and a demoralised team, where do you start?

Jerry Sternin, working for Save the Children, was faced with a parallel question. When asked to open a new office in Vietnam to tackle malnutrition, he knew he had a problem. The Foreign Minister told him frostily: 'You have six months to make a difference.'

Sternin knew the realities of childhood malnutrition, a dynamic of poverty, sanitation, and nutrition. But he couldn't tackle the fundamental infrastructure behind these problems in six months.

So he travelled to rural villages to meet groups of mothers, setting up teams to weigh and measure the children in the villages. His question 'Do you find very poor children who are bigger and healthier than others?' met the answer 'yes'.

Sternin searched in each community for the 'bright spots', the successful activities that would be worth replicating. He found practical suggestions that made a difference. For instance, 'bright spot mothers' were feeding their children four times a day – using the same amount of food as other mothers, but spreading it across four rather than two servings – a tactic that made it easier for children to digest the food.

Because Sternin is a smart guy, he didn't turn his findings into a manual: 'The Five Rules to Fight Malnutrition'. Instead, he shared his results village by village, in cooking classes, to allow the community to work through and implement the changes. The programme went on to reach 2.2 million Vietnamese people, with 65 per cent of the children becoming better nourished.

When we're faced with the need to change but don't have the answers or a budget to implement solutions, beginning with the bright spots is a good start.

11.6   Speak to the Elephant as Well as the Rider

John Kotter's *The Heart of Change* summarises the results of 130 companies in the implementation of successful change. Kotter makes the point that the typical change programme focuses on strategy, systems, and structure and misses the 'core of the matter . . . behaviour change happens by speaking to people's feelings'.

Jonathan Haidt uses the metaphor of the Elephant and the Rider to describe the way in which our brains work. Our emotional side is the Elephant, and the rational is the Rider. The rational ego of the Rider sits atop the Elephant holding the reins, apparently in control. But the Rider's position is precarious, because the Rider is much smaller than the Elephant. If the Elephant disagrees with the Rider about which direction to go in, the Rider is going to lose.

Our Elephant – our emotional and instinctive side – looks for a quick pay-off that feels good now. The Rider, aware of the drawbacks of instant gratification, is concerned to think rationally and plan for the future. But the Elephant isn't always the bad guy. The Elephant's emotions of love and compassion and sympathy and loyalty are positive forces. And it is the emotions of the Elephant, its energy and drive, which get things done. While the rational Rider is spinning the wheels of overanalysis and overthinking, the Elephant pushes on.

Change works when it speaks to both the Elephant and the Rider.

If you're presenting a proposal for change, go beyond the number-crunching logic of cost–benefit analysis to appeal to other people's emotions and feelings. Instead of the typical sequence the Rider follows of Analyse–Think–Change, shift to a message that will resonate with the Elephant: See–Feel–Change.

Do

11.7 How Good Is Good?

Good is good. But as Jim Collins points out in *Good to Great*, 'good is the enemy of greatness'. Good makes us feel we've made it, and when we slip into comfortable complacency, it holds us back from the trajectory to greatness.

- Are you good or great?
- Review the range of your knowledge, expertise, talents, and skills to identify two or three themes that are 'good'. These are your current strengths, strengths that if developed could become areas of exceptional performance.
- Note what they are, and what you could do to turn 'good' into 'great'. Is it simply a programme of continued practice to develop greater proficiency? Or can you accelerate the process?
- What tactics will you use to go from 'good' to 'great'?

11.8 Develop a T-Shaped Mind

Focus on developing excellence within your professional expertise. But it's worth remembering that pioneers in innovation go beyond in-depth mastery of their specialist area to keep a curious and direct interest about other fields. This is innovation. In Isaiah Berlin's famous classification part hedgehog (those who know one thing and know it well) and part fox (those who know many small things and are flexible in 'ad hocery').

If you want to catalyse excellence, maintain a breadth of perspective to complement your professional focus. This could be:

- Initiating dialogue with people from other disciplines with different interests.
- Attending conferences, training events, and programmes in other fields.
- Reading widely to keep in touch with overall social, political, and economic trends.
- Extending your online social networks to participate in a range of different interest groups.

Ask yourself:

- How well developed is your T-shaped mind?
- What do you plan to do to develop it further?

11.9 From What to What?

When you're planning a significant change, it's a useful exercise to ask yourself or the team you're working with: 'From what to what?'

In this exercise, think of a change you want to make, identifying the current situation and the future desired state. Now write pairs of words that summarise 'from what to what?'

- What words are being used?
- How aspirational is the future you describe?
- How insightful are the words about the current situation?
- What do these words indicate about the size of the gap?

Review the pairs of words you have generated, comparing and contrasting the differences between current and future. If you don't feel energised about the change that lies ahead, you might want to revisit your pairing of words.

Note the outcomes of this exercise. Did it help move you from abstract thinking about change in theory to make the process more grounded?

In a Nutshell: Change to Implement Excellence

Is good the enemy of the great? Why is change – incremental and radical – important in leadership life?

This chapter introduced six things you should know about innovation and change. How does the culture and climate of your work area encourage or discourage innovation?

You discovered that in planning change, it helps to start with the bright spots, those successful activities worth replicating. In implementing change, communication with colleagues should appeal to the 'Elephant', not just the 'Rider'. Here we engage with others' feelings and motivations.

The chapter concluded with an exercise to help you move from abstract to concrete thinking about your desired changes.

12

Recognising Personality Types

Dental professionals meet a large number of patients every day, so it is important for us to understand different perspectives, ask ourselves why people behave as they do, and know how to communicate with different personalities.

> *It's not what you eat between Christmas and New Year that causes weight gain. It's what you eat between New Year and Christmas that is the challenge.*

> *Every person has three characters: that which they exhibit, that which they have, and that which they think they have.*
>
> Alphonse Karr

In this chapter you will learn about:

- The realities of human nature, including unknown intentions, selfish altruism, and the need for reassurance.
- Three levels to know someone, including personality traits, personal concerns, and understanding life stories.
- A simple lens on human understanding, and personality types including the 'get it done', 'get it right', and 'get along' approach.
- Reading personality with one good question about traits.
- Personality and its impact on communication: Analyticals, Amiables, Expressives, and Drivers.
- Those you need to understand but don't.
- Personality and team dynamics.

Overview

> *The shoe that fits one person pinches another; there is no recipe for living that suits all cases.*
>
> Carl Jung

Leadership Skills for Dental Professionals: Begin Well to Finish Well, First Edition.
Raman Bedi, Andrew Munro and Mark Keane.
© 2022 John Wiley & Sons Ltd. Published 2022 by John Wiley & Sons Ltd.

People have much in common, but we are also different. Understanding these differences and their implications will help us become better professionals. If we don't acknowledge and understand these fairly deep-seated and fundamental differences, we will make life more difficult than it needs to be – for our patients, our colleagues, and ourselves as practitioners.

We will also be able to relate to people, influence people, and lead people more efficiently to better oral health if we are aware of different personality types. This chapter will help you to explore this.

Think

12.1   The Realities of Human Nature

> *Science changes but human nature does not.*
>
> Sherwin Nuland

As we saw in Chapter 9, humans have different and distinctive talents and strengths, which are shaped by our varying histories, backgrounds, and experiences. You will remember from Section 9.2 some generalisations about other people:

- **Most people don't care all that much about you**.
- **Most intentions are unknown**.
- **Selfish altruism explains a lot**.
- **Bad memories**.
- **Emotions call the shots**.
- **People need reassurance**.

In our interactions with others, we walk a fine line between cynicism that assumes the worst of others and naivety that adopts an idealistic view of human perfection. We may quickly be disappointed by other people's behaviour.

We optimise our impact when we start with a positive view of others, but don't forget the realities of human nature.

- Is cynicism holding you back?

12.2   Three Levels of Knowing Someone

What does it mean to know someone?

There are three levels in getting to know your patients (Figure 12.1):

- The first relies on the **broad description of personality traits**. Some people are agreeable, others assertive or moody, and so on. This isn't a bad start if it helps us adapt our approach to the different types of individual we will encounter, but this level does not provide a comprehensive understanding.
- The second level moves on from the mapping of personality dimensions to **appreciate personal concerns**: how people define themselves with reference to the roles they play,

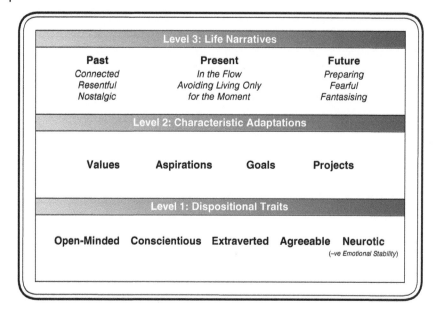

Figure 12.1   Knowing your patients and colleagues.

the skills they value, the interests that make them passionate, and the goals they have for the future.

- The third level of 'getting to know' people is to **understand the life story** that individuals construct to connect their past, present, and anticipated future. This is how individuals make sense of their lives; at this level we gain a deeper understanding of their fears and concerns, priorities and pressures, aspirations and dreams. Understanding a patient's life story will help us to be sensitive to it.

This third level of insight is gained through our willingness to listen to others' life stories and share our own life narrative. If self-disclosure is difficult for us, we may also find it difficult to understand others.

We can't get to know every team member or colleague at the third level, but we can only really understand other people if we are also prepared to share something of our own life story.

12.3   A Simple Lens of Human Understanding

> *Ninety per cent of the world's woes come from people not knowing themselves, their abilities, their frailties, and even their real virtues.*
>
> Sidney J Harris

There is no shortage of personality frameworks and systems, ranging from the simple (and simplistic) to the complex that are impractical to apply in practice life.

Here are types of personality you may see in your colleagues (Figure 12.2):

- **Get It Done** is a combination of High Task and High Aggressive. At best, this is a directive approach that is quick to spot problems, overcome challenges, and implement

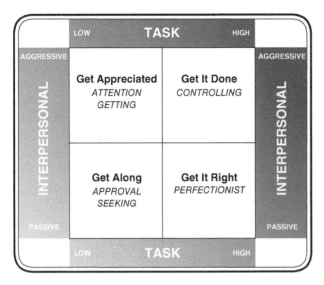

Figure 12.2 Personality types.

solutions. At worst, others can find this approach overly demanding, intimidating, and want to maintain a distance from us. Alternatively, our 'just do it' outlook may encourage others to take expedient short-cuts, with damaging consequences for the long term.

- **Get It Right** combines High Task and High Passive, which attends to the detail of work activity and is conscientious in tackling problems in a systematic and methodical way. Here we work to high standards. But there is a risk that we become overwhelmed, taking on too much in accommodating others' expectations.
- **Get Along** is a combination of Low Task and High Passive, which is an agreeable approach that values positive relationships and maintains interpersonal harmony. This is the outlook that, at best, makes for an enjoyable work environment. At worst, it is an easy-going work style that avoids the difficult issues that might open up conflict and allows problems to persist.
- **Get Appreciated** combines Low Task and High Aggressive, and results in an outlook in which we look to take the lead and provide direction to others. Here, at best, we provide inspiration for our patients and colleagues. At worst, our need for status and recognition (too much 'me' and not enough 'we') annoys others and becomes counter-productive.

In the Do section of this chapter there will be an opportunity to review your own personality and how it might shape your approach. But at this stage, use this lens as a simple way to identify your typical operating style and also think about the colleagues you work with.

12.4 Reading Personality – One Good Question

We sharpen our interpersonal skills and optimise our overall effectiveness if we can read and understand the behaviour of others. This isn't a strategy of labelling and stereotyping based on first impressions. Human nature and behaviour are complex and an open mind, curiosity to learn, and a willingness to update our judgements make for better tactics than the application of any one 'secret' to understanding others in five minutes.

We can use idiosyncratic ways to make sense of others' personalities: check out their pets and the names they call them; read their car and bumper stickers; look at their music or book collection and other stuff in their homes. Or we can ask a simple question.

If you want to know if a person displays a specific personality trait, just ask them if they think other people often display that trait.

When people rate others, for example as kind, they're more likely to rate themselves as kind. Seeing others as having specific positive traits identifies their own positive traits. And this question works for darker personality traits. If we think that others are manipulative, for example, the chances are that we are more likely to be manipulative ourselves.

We understand others and their personality when we listen to find out how they talk about others' personalities.

And if that does not work, ask the person out to a restaurant and see how they treat the waiting staff.

12.5   Personality and Its Impact on Communication

There are many reasons why communication is a challenge, even in relatively small work teams. Between the giver and the receiver there are many opportunities for the signal to get lost in transmission, or for the signal to be misinterpreted, with unintended consequences.

Personality differences play a major factor in accounting for communication breakdown, and help explain why communication can be downright impossible with some patients but effortless with others.

Here are four personality styles:

- **Analyticals** are patients who like data, facts, and information. For Analyticals, detail is their preference and communication should be precise and well defined. They respond well to lists of pros and cons.
- **Amiables** are cheerful and helpful types who like to be involved in discussions and are keen to provide their support. For Amiables, conversations are an opportunity to build relationships and ensure there is a consensus. Communication with Amiables may be an interesting but meandering process.
- **Expressives** are enthusiastic and extraverted types who throw themselves into activity, keen to have their voice heard. Expressives enjoy communication, but mainly their own, and may not listen actively to others. It is important you ensure that they have understood your messages fully.
- **Drivers** look for results quickly, keen to get to grips with problems and make progress against goals. Communication for Drivers is fast, direct, and to the point, but there may be less check-in for understanding. Also be careful of how fast they want results – is this realistic? They may be disappointed!

Even with only these four communication styles, it is easy to see how misunderstandings emerge.

The Driver issues an overall directive, but the Analytical finds this confusing. They want more detail on the specific requirement.

The Driver then becomes frustrated at the lack of progress and repeats the original demand, but with more urgency.

The Analytical – still looking for clarity on exactly what is required – becomes increasingly puzzled. And so on.

The Amiable wants to raise an issue, but the Expressive interrupts and goes off at a tangent. The Amiable decides to let the problem go, and the Expressive assumes that the problem has disappeared.

Of course, the problem remains unresolved, but becomes bigger. And at some point the Expressive gets agitated, asking why no one mentioned it.

Check your dominant communication style to ask yourself:

- What are the strengths that I bring to effective communication?
- What specific risks might be associated with this approach?
- Which other styles do I find most difficult?
- What tactics do I use to manage communication processes with these styles?
- Is there a dominant communication style within my workplace? Is it working positively for the work group and for clients?
- Or is it creating problems of coordination? How?

Do

12.6   Who I Need to Understand but Don't

Take a few minutes to think of a person who is important to you, but where the relationship doesn't quite work. It's not necessarily a bad relationship, but it is not one that works well, and if it were to improve, your working life would be better, easier, and happier.

- Who is the individual?
- How does this individual make you feel? Use three or four words to describe how you typically feel with this individual (e.g. nervous, impatient, baffled).
- How do you think you make this person feel?
- How would you describe the person's personality using the Big Five model of personality (see Level 1: Dispositional Traits in Figure 12.1)?
- Given your own personality, how might this explain the dynamics of your relationship? Can you identify the reasons for any difficulty?
- Given your personality, what could you do more or less of to improve this relationship?

12.7   Personality and Team Dynamics

Personality also affects the way teams operate. Look at your own team and ask:

- Is it effective?
- Do you have what it takes to be a good team member?
- Or are you and the personality style you bring to the practice a factor in any challenges the team faces?

When we choose team members for work, technical and professional skills are of course critical. But it is also useful to think about personality and its impact within an effective team. Some leaders – particularly of the narcissistic variety – pick team members who are like them. In the short term it might make for personal chemistry, but over time this approach undermines diversity and gives rise to counter-productive groupthink.

- Which personality styles do you think a dental practice team needs more of or less of to enhance its overall effectiveness?

In a Nutshell: Recognising Personality Types

Recognising personality types will help you as a leader to understand different perspectives, why people behave as they do, and how to communicate with different personalities.

First, what are the realities of human nature? What does it mean to know someone? This chapter reviewed three levels of personality to go from a superficial description to a genuine understanding of the individual.

Reading personality draws your focus to one good question for valuable personality insights.

Understanding personality and its impact on communication helps you identify four personality styles for improved engagement with colleagues. The chapter also encouraged you to reflect on the strengths and limitations of your dominant communication style.

13

Get Fluent in Body Language

When you see a new patient, first impressions are important. A key component of that impression will be your body language. The body language of dental professionals is important in gaining the confidence of your patients.

> *Tina, we've gotten some complaints about your hostile behavior. At a recent meeting, you crossed your arms. That is unacceptable body language.*
> *Tina: Maybe I was cold!*
>
> Scott Adams

In this chapter you will learn about:

- Five myths of body language, including that 93 per cent of body language is communication, liars don't make eye contact, and crossed arms mean resistance.
- The body language of trust and respect, including how to develop trust, projecting happiness, and hand gestures.
- The body language of the alpha leader, including smiling less, interrupting, and switching eye contact.
- The 15 most common body language blunders, including slouching, exaggerated nodding, intense eye contact, and how to smile authentically.
- Body language and cultural differences, including personal space, handshaking, and agreement.
- Lying, including confusion with anxiety, pitch of voice, communication patterns, and the relevance of context.
- Evaluating how well you read other people and their non-verbal body language.
- Tactics for more effective body language, including awareness of what you communicate, making discomfort signals, and matching body language with words.

Leadership Skills for Dental Professionals: Begin Well to Finish Well, First Edition.
Raman Bedi, Andrew Munro and Mark Keane.
© 2022 John Wiley & Sons Ltd. Published 2022 by John Wiley & Sons Ltd.

Overview

> *There are four ways, and only four ways, in which we have contact with the world. We are evaluated and classified by these four contacts: what we do, how we look, what we say, and how we say it.*
>
> Dale Carnegie

What people say is not always what they mean or are feeling. This is not always about deception, where there is inconsistency between intentions and words. The gap between what we say and what we mean or feel can result from many different factors, and can sometimes be out of fear, shame, embarrassment, pride, or anger.

Understanding body language and reading other people's is not about the science of manipulation. If we understand our own body language and its impact, and improve how we interpret others' non-verbal behaviour, we become more skilled in understanding the intentions and motivations of our friends and colleagues, and are better able to adapt our approach to optimise our impact. And if we are not aware of how others are coming across to us and how we are coming across to them, we are missing a large part of human interaction.

This chapter covers the domain of body language and some of the associated myths and realities, to provide another lens and skill set to improve your effectiveness as a professional.

Think

13.1   Five Myths about Body Language

Because body language has been the focus of those with a particular interest in influence, it is probably unsurprising that a few myths have emerged.

13.1.1   Body Language is 93 Percent of Communication

A classic study is often misquoted as 'the total impact of a message is based on: 7% words used; 38% tone of voice, volume, rate of speech, vocal pitch; 55% facial expressions, hand gestures, postures, and other forms of body language'. But this is not what the research revealed. Yes, non-verbal communication matters, but if we rely on it too much, we forget the importance of the content of our message.

13.1.2   Liars Don't Make Eye Contact

While some liars find it difficult to lie while looking you in the eyes, most liars, probably the most skilful, 'prove' that they are not lying by holding eye contact and holding it too long.

13.1.3   Crossed Arms Mean Resistance

If someone crosses their arms it might indicate disagreement or opposition. It may also be a signal of concentration and persistence; or that there has been a drop in room temperature. But given that most people believe this myth, be careful when folding your arms in conversation, particularly when meeting people for the first time.

13.1.4 Eye Direction Correlates with Lying

This idea, much loved by adherents of neurolinguistic programming (NLP), suggests that looking to the right indicates lying, while looking to the left suggests truth telling. Nevertheless, it is now known to be false.

13.1.5 Using Body Language to Make a Positive Impression is Inauthentic

Of course, there is nothing worse than an NLP novice who has discovered the mirroring technique and attempts to mimic our every move. This rightly strikes us as false and contrived. But working on our own impact and improving our understanding of interpersonal exchanges seem highly worthwhile goals.

13.2 The Body Language of Trust and Respect

Leaders are trusted and respected when they:

- Project happiness rather than frustration, anxiety, or hostility.
- Display positive language. When sitting, it's better to lean back slightly rather than forward, and to keep your arms away from the side of your body.
- Use hand gestures to emphasise their arguments. Arguments about expansion and growth should be accompanied by hands that move away from one another. And arguments about problems and contraction are associated with hands that move towards one another.
- Trim thick, bushy eyebrows; apparently thick brows are associated with hostility!

All of these points probably need to be taken with a pinch of salt. But it's still worth checking if your body language is enhancing or damaging your credibility in working with different individuals and groups.

13.3 The Body Language of the Alpha Leader

Much has been written about the body language of the alpha leader. Some of the specifics include the following:

- **Smiling less**. This is not saying that we want to avoid the genuine warmth of a friendly personality who is keen to make contact. Rather, if we want to project confidence and authority, we should avoid the awkward smile of the nervous subordinate.
- **Interrupting**. Of course, interrupting can be bad manners arising out of a lack of respect for others. It can also be having the confidence to interject when a colleague is talking too much and others in the group are becoming bored or unhappy. Or it is sometimes the willingness to stop someone in their tracks if their nervousness is taking them into an unhelpful ramble and making them even more nervous.

- **Switching eye contact**. Alpha leaders hold eye contact when they are speaking but look away when others speak to them. Again this can be bad manners, motivated more by power games than by genuine leadership. But if our gaze rests for too long on others when they speak, we may find that they assume greater influence than they deserve.
- **Standing still**. If we fidget, pace the room, and hop around, we are signalling our anxiety to others, and may be at risk of undermining our authority.
- **Holding the head still**. Nodding and bobbing signal an edgy agreeableness that can make others feel tense. It is a gesture of submissiveness that affects our ability to take the lead and exert our authority.

Don't overdo the body language of the alpha leader and embark on games like the 'power handshake' or silence to make other people uncomfortable. But be alert to any behaviours that might weaken your authority and of the tactics others may use with you in interpersonal encounters in an attempt to overplay their authority at your expense.

13.4   The 15 Most Common Body Language Blunders

What you do speaks so loud that I cannot hear what you say.

Ralph Waldo Emerson

If you want to finesse your skills in reading body language, a good starting point is to avoid the mistakes that people commonly make:

- **Slouching**: a sign of disrespect, and a signal that we are bored and would rather be somewhere else. Sit straight to engage others.
- **Exaggerated gestures**: a form of histrionics by which we stretch the truth. Small, controlled, and open gestures indicate confidence in our position and that we have nothing to hide.
- **Clock watching**: an indicator of impatience and a signal that our time matters more to us than to others, and that we are way more important than them.
- **Turning away**: a sign that we are uninterested, uncomfortable, or suspicious of others. When we lean in towards someone, we indicate our full attention to engaging in the conversation.
- **Crossed arms**: not always a sign of defensiveness, but others can interpret this gesture as a barrier to open communication.
- **Inconsistency**: incongruence between what we say and the expressions we use to say it. This is either just weird and confuses others, or they suspect we are being deceptive in some way.
- **Exaggerated nodding**: indicates we are anxious for approval from others, or they may think we are agreeing to something when we are not.
- **Fidgeting**: tapping of fingers, fixing of hair, and scratching of our body parts, which all signal that we are anxious and distracted.
- **Avoiding eye contact**: either we are fearful and anxious, or we are implying that we have something to hide. It is a signal that others dislike.

- **Intense eye contact**: a scary action that others will view as aggressive and intimidating.
- **Eye rolling**: perhaps one of the worst mistakes to make. We are sending out a strong statement of a lack of respect for the other person.
- **Scowling**: variations of an unhappy face, all of which indicate a negative message that others find off-putting and upsetting.
- **A weak handshake**: the extreme opposite, a bone-crushing handshake that seeks to intimidate, is to be avoided, but a weak handshake will be interpreted as lacking in confidence and authority.
- **Clenched fists**: a signal that we are not receptive to others' viewpoints and that we are preparing for an argument.
- **Getting too close**: mismanaging others' personal space, which makes them uncomfortable.

13.5   How to Smile

A warm smile is the universal language of kindness.

William Arthur Ward

Smiling is generally viewed as a good thing in social interaction. In contrast, a frown or scowl is no doubt a bad thing in building the kind of rapport that facilitates open communication. Research indicates the importance of smiling, in particular:

- An **authentic smile**: the 'Duchenne' smile, in which the corners of the mouth turn up and the skin around the corners of the eyes crinkles, in contrast to the grimace of the perfunctory smile.
- A **long-onset smile**: a smile that appears slowly rather than switches on immediately.
- **Congruence** with other cues, e.g. eye movement, head tilt, and gestures.

Smiles that build trust are revealed through the eyes, emerge slowly, and are accompanied by positive body language. If you're not a natural at smiling, be careful that your attempts aren't viewed as false and insincere.

13.6   Body Language and Cultural Differences

In conversations there is often a difference between what we say and what we mean. Consequently, the listener interprets the meaning based not on what we actually say, but on how we say it and on our body language. Interactions with other cultures can be even more problematic when we not only speak a different language, but also use a different body language: how we greet others, how we sit or stand, our facial expressions, our clothes, hairstyle, tone of voice, eye movements, how we listen, how we breathe, how close we stand to others, and how we touch others can all vary depending on where we were born and brought up.

In general, some facial expressions are universally recognised: happiness, sadness, fear, disgust, surprise, anger, and boredom. Smiling is recognised around the world and is always a good way of breaking the ice when in doubt.

Gestures cannot be taken in isolation. Rubbing your nose can be an indication of lying – but it can also mean you've got an itchy nose. The most reliable indicators come from reading clusters of gestures, like reading all the words of a sentence. Look also for congruence between the words that are said, the way they are said, and the body language exhibited.

Eye contact is regarded as a sign of sincerity and honesty in Western countries. Someone who doesn't look you in the eye can appear shifty or seem to be hiding something. On the other hand, someone staring at you for too long can appear rude or hostile. However, some cultures regard the avoidance of eye contact as a sign of respect, while others will maintain a look for longer than you may feel comfortable with.

Personal space is generally regarded as a four-foot circle around you. Those you are on close terms with can enter the circle, but if others attempt to do so you feel uncomfortable. Cultures vary in the amount of space they regard as normal.

Handshaking is a widely used greeting. A firm handshake is often regarded as honest, forthright, and confident, while a limp one is seen as wishy-washy and weak. You cannot apply this interpretation to all cultures, however. In Arab countries people shake hands more frequently but less firmly. The right hand will always be used, as the left hand is regarded as unclean because of its association with bodily functions. Japanese people bow on meeting rather than shaking hands, and the deeper the bow the more respect is being shown.

Agreement is signalled by shaking the head sideways in countries such as Greece and Turkey; in other countries nodding the head means no. In Japan, the word 'no' may be avoided to prevent causing offence or loss of face. Japanese people are more likely to lower their eyes and say 'yes, but' or give alternatives.

Each culture has its own set of non-verbal communication that we should be aware of in building relationships of respect and trust.

13.7 Lying

Given the prevalence of lying, it isn't surprising that we've developed a range of lie-detection tactics. As Richard Wiseman points out, some of these measures have been extreme. In the 'red hot poker' test, the suspected liar is asked to lick a red hot poker, the rationale being that someone who is innocent would have enough saliva in their mouth to prevent burning. However, the guilty liar's high level of anxiety would dry their mouth.

Typical indicators of anxiety – avoidance of eye contact; shifting from foot to foot; sweaty hands; covering the mouth with hands; long and rambling answers – aren't very good lie detectors. Remember that everyone is different. Some people's natural behaviour (typically the nervous introvert) can appear shifty, and others (the stable extravert) can come across as honest. Don't jump to conclusions.

So what does indicate lying?

- **Pitch of voice**. Of all the tell-tale signs, the pitch of someone's voice is probably the most reliable indicator that they are being less than honest. Liars have a slightly higher pitch of voice than truth-tellers.
- **Less movement and more pauses.** Because lying is cognitively demanding (having to remember previous lies, reading the recipient's body language, embedding lies

within a plausible account), liars tend to do what we all do when we have to think hard. So liars don't gesture too much, they repeat the same phrases, and they pause for longer. Question a potential liar with more demanding questions and these signals will increase.

- **Communication patterns**. Liars give shorter and less detailed answers, and they minimise the personal ('me', 'mine', 'I' words).

Although we think that visual cues – body language – provide a revealing insight into possible lying, in fact vocal and verbal cues – what is said and how it is said – are much more reliable indicators. And if you're still unsure whether someone is lying, ask them to send the message through in an email. Liars know that emails are recorded and archived and that their falsehoods can be identified.

13.8   Context Is Critical

We improve our skills in reading other people's body language when we remember the importance of context. If we understand the interplay of situational factors, we avoid jumping to the kind of conclusions that will lead to mistaken interpretations of others' intentions and motivations.

If a colleague has crossed their arms, what does this indicate? It could be that:

- They are upset and angry with you.
- The conversational topic is not one they like.
- They have suddenly remembered an argument they had with their partner that morning.
- They have spotted that you have spinach stuck on a tooth and aren't sure how to tell you.
- The heating has stopped working and they are cold.

Our interpersonal exchanges take place within a context that reflect the dynamics of our behaviour, other's behaviour (and what else is going in their lives), and the situation and environment.

If we think that someone's body language is indicating they are uncomfortable, we can always ask a question in a straightforward and genuine manner: 'Is everything OK?' It might be a simpler tactic than misreading their body language and drawing the wrong conclusion.

Do

13.9   How Well Do You Read Other People?

Test your skill at reading non-verbal behaviour by watching a reality TV programme with the sound turned off. Can you easily work out the interpersonal dynamics at play?

If you can identify who is most and least popular, assertive, confident, or competitive, then you are deploying a key skill in reading body language.

13.10   Tactics for More Effective Body Language

To change your body language, you must first be aware of it. Notice how you sit, how you stand, how you use your hands and legs, what you do while talking to someone.

Be aware of what your body is communicating and make the effort to mute any discomfort signals. Matching your body language to your words will provide the consistency that others value: when you are relaxed and self-assured, but also when you are uncomfortable. It is incongruence that others find difficult.

You might want to practise in front of a mirror. Yes, it will be slightly strange at first, but it's very safe; after all, no one is watching you. Alternatively, close your eyes and visualise how you would stand and sit to feel confident, open, and relaxed, or whatever you want to communicate. Then try it out.

Or ask for feedback from a trusted colleague. What do they see you doing in your interactions within the dental team and with patients? Here, park any defensiveness on your part, and be willing to listen and hear the feedback.

In a Nutshell: Get Fluent in Body Language

What people say may be different to what they mean or feel. This chapter has focused on body language and outlined a few myths and realities.

Fifteen of the most common body language blunders are highlighted, but no examination of body language would be complete without reference to cultural differences.

Do you know how to spot a liar? It's easier said than done, but this chapter will help.

The chapter concluded its look at fluency in body language with two exercises designed to improve your skill in reading non-verbal behaviour and ensuring your own is congruent.

14

Be Assertive

Providing dental care embraces so many aspects of one's life. Our patients have multiple expectations of us. It is important to understand how we can overcome shyness and embarrassment, be competent in public speaking, be assertive in dental practice, manage our mistakes, and of course understand the art of an apology.

> *Confidence is knowing who you are and not changing it a bit because of someone's version of reality is not your reality.*
>
> Shannon L. Alder

In this chapter you will learn about:

- Evaluating whether your thinking is unassertive, including not saying what you are thinking, interpretation of a lack of response, and believing that resolution can be achieved by not saying anything.
- Overcoming shyness, including a weak self-image, preoccupation with ourselves, and self-defeating phrases.
- Dealing with criticism, including acknowledging it as progress, taking it in your stride, and accepting praise and criticism evenly.
- Avoiding embarrassment, including acknowledging that you are rarely in the spotlight and understanding that your shortcomings are likely not noticeable.
- Managing anxiety, including accepting worry as a life fact and controlling your worry time.
- Managing mistakes as an indicator of assertiveness, including seeing mistakes as a measure of progress, admitting honest mistakes, and stopping mistakes getting worse.
- Assertiveness and the art of the apology, including avoiding excuses, apologising with grace, responsibility, and restitution.
- Voice tips, including how to use your voice well, pitch, pauses, and passion.
- Presentation fundamentals, including how to avoid obvious mistakes, failure to research the audience, and asserting unsupported opinions.
- How to be assertive, including fogging to stay calm in the face of criticism and DESC scripting to understand what is happening and the consequences.

Leadership Skills for Dental Professionals: Begin Well to Finish Well, First Edition.
Raman Bedi, Andrew Munro and Mark Keane.
© 2022 John Wiley & Sons Ltd. Published 2022 by John Wiley & Sons Ltd.

Overview

With passive behaviour, l lose, you win. With aggressive behaviour, I win, you lose. And with assertive behaviour, I win, you win.

Being assertive is not about being loud and domineering, but about resisting those who try to dominate or manipulate us, enabling us to speak up and take more control in important situations. We can say 'yes' and mean 'yes', and say 'no' and mean 'no'. We can speak freely without fearing conflict. We feel entitled to be who we are and express our views.

Assertiveness is important to our professional lives. It ensures that our interests are understood by others. It helps us stick up for our colleagues who may be being treated badly. It is also important in how we manage difficult patient relationships, as well as providing the kind of challenge that finds ways to keep improving our professional practice. Nevertheless, it is important not to confuse assertiveness with the arrogance of abusing our power and authority, or the aggression that is the expression of any negative emotions.

Being assertive is not always easy, and it is more difficult for some individuals than others. This chapter is about the tactics of assertiveness to manage situations where we feel less assertive.

Think

14.1   Is Your Thinking Unassertive?

Our levels of assertiveness are shaped by the beliefs we hold, about ourselves, other people, and how the world works. And if we don't recognise the impact of our thoughts, we may find assertiveness a challenge. Unassertive thoughts include:

- 'I can't say what I'm feeling because I don't want to burden others with my problems.'
- 'It is rude to state what I want.'
- 'If I assert myself I might upset others and ruin the relationship.'
- 'I will create an embarrassing situation if I say what I think.'
- 'If someone says no, it means they don't like me.'
- 'If I keep quiet, things will sort of work out in the end.'

If we shift our mind-set to remember our rights, our thoughts might switch to a more assertive position. We have the right to:

- Express our feelings, beliefs, and opinions.
- Say yes and no.
- Change our mind.
- Disagree with others if we think they are wrong.
- Say 'I don't understand'.
- Decline to take on responsibility for others' problems.
- Make reasonable requests of others.
- Set our own priorities and manage our time.
- Be listened to and taken seriously.
- Make mistakes and feel comfortable admitting to them.

14.2   Overcoming Shyness

Scientists have found the gene for shyness. They would have found it years ago, but it was hiding behind a couple of other genes.

Jonathan Katz

It's part of the reality of personality differences that some individuals relish social interaction, and others find the experience more difficult. In fact, 40 per cent of people describe themselves as shy. But when shyness becomes severe and we avoid social situations, it can have a major impact on our professional success. Productive time is wasted in the worry about forthcoming social encounters.

Shyness may lead to:

- **A weak self-image**: we've not yet worked out who we are and feel we haven't become a dynamic professional that others will find interesting.
- **A preoccupation with ourselves**: a heightened self-consciousness in which we become acutely aware of what we're doing and fear that others will think badly of us.
- **Labelling**: because we tell ourselves we're shy, we think we must be shy and we behave in ways that confirm our shyness.

There are some tactics you can use to overcome shyness:

- **Identify the benefits** of the social situation ahead of you and how it can be a positive experience. Don't allow short-term worries to lead to you losing sight of the longer-term gains.
- Always **look your best**. Bad personal hygiene, poor grooming, and lack of dress sense can make us shy. Look the part to project yourself well.
- **Act as if you are a confident person**. However tough it feels, manage your posture, body language, and speech to project confidence. Smile, and smile as if you mean it. Don't compound your shyness with a demeanour that suggests you want to be somewhere else. Others will assume you do want to be somewhere else and avoid you.
- **Watch for self-defeating phrases** such as 'I'm boring', or 'I don't have anything interesting to say'. These phrases will make you boring because no one will want to talk to you.
- **Manage the fear of rejection** by thinking 'So what?' Would it be that bad if no one talked to you for a while?
- **Concentrate on others** within the social situation and avoid focusing on your own feelings. The world is not looking at you; most people are too busy thinking about themselves. Rather than focusing on your own awkwardness in social situations, focus on other people and what they have to say. Encourage others to talk about themselves. As you're conversing, ask: 'What is it about this person that I like?'
- **Manage your breathing**. When we're anxious, our body and breathing patterns change, making us even more tense. Use relaxation techniques to control your breathing.

Shyness isn't a disorder with a cure. It's a life pattern that has built up and been reinforced. And you can develop strategies and tactics to change this pattern and become more socially confident.

14.3   Having a Thick or Thin Skin: Dealing with Criticism

The best way to avoid criticism is to establish a reputation for being irrational and belligerent at the slightest excuse.

Dilbert

I defy anyone to tell me that she or he has ever felt indifferent, let alone uplifted, enriched, cheered up, or enhanced when put on the receiving end of a blast of criticism.

Sydney B. Simon

Like the physical immune system that defends our bodies against illness, our mind is alert to protect us from potential unhappiness. And like the physical system, which must strike a balance between spotting and eliminating dangerous invaders while respecting the body's integrity, our psychological immune system must find a way of defending us, but not so well that our defensiveness damages our interests.

If our psychological immune system is underactive, life's slings and arrows overwhelm us. We become rejected, demoralised, and depressed. But with an overactive system we become detached from reality. Certain of our own brilliance and convinced that the world is engaged in a vast conspiracy to attack us, we lose touch with reality and retreat into neuroticism or paranoia.

We all hate criticism, particularly when we think we are doing a good job. It can bring out our worst emotions and if allowed to fester undermines our performance. On the other hand, criticism can be constructive when it highlights a problem, clears the air, or just motivates. But it can be difficult to tell the difference between positive and negative criticism.

There are a couple of ways to deal with criticism.

14.3.1   Most Criticism Indicates Progress

Criticism is something we can avoid easily by saying nothing, doing nothing, and being nothing. The absence of any personal criticism indicates a lack of drive to achieve anything new or different. Anyone who attempts to make a difference will meet some kind of opposition. Criticism is difficult, but if you know how to manage it you can deal assertively with others' aggressive put-downs. But don't be defensive in responding to every perceived slight. Accept that some criticism you need to 'take on the chin'. Learn from it and shift your approach.

How you respond to criticism can be a constructive or destructive experience. Where constructive, it takes the form of feedback and you can learn from it, choose to ignore it or assert your viewpoint. Criticism can have some justification, but if it is delivered in a hostile way or is completely unjustified, it is destructive. Realise that it's not just about you: the critic may be like that to everyone, may be going through a difficult period, or may be jealous of your achievements. You can:

- Take it in your stride, staying calm and listening without reaction.
- Consider points that will help you and learn from them.
- View both praise and criticism evenly. Try not to get too excited when you are praised and adopt the same approach when criticised.

14.3.2 Think Like Buddha

A man interrupted one of Buddha's lectures with a flood of abuse. Buddha waited until he had finished and then asked him, 'If a man offered a gift to another but the gift was declined, to whom would the gift belong?'

'To the one who offered it,' said the man.

'Then,' said the Buddha, 'I decline to accept your abuse and request you to keep it for yourself.'

Simply don't accept the gift of criticism. You don't have to. Then it still belongs to the person who offered it.

14.4 Avoiding Embarrassment

> *The 18/40/60 Rule: 'When you're 18, you worry about what everybody is thinking of you; when you're 40, you don't give a damn what anybody thinks of you; when you're 60, you realise nobody's been thinking about you at all.'*

14.4.1 Get Past the Point of Embarrassment

The fear of embarrassment, that sense of social shame when we blunder, commit some gaffe, or create awkwardness, is a major barrier to progress. Don't let it hold you back. If you are easily embarrassed, then say so when you're managing any differences and disagreements: 'I don't know why I am embarrassed in saying this. But I am. But it is important to me to say it so you understand my views. . .'

Don't allow others to exploit your embarrassment. Acknowledge it and use it to your advantage.

14.4.2 You're Rarely in the Spotlight

In one piece of research, students were asked to put on T-shirts before being introduced to a group. The downside: emblazoned on the T-shirts was a large photograph of Barry Manilow. The students joined, then left the group after a few minutes. They were asked to estimate the percentage of the group who had noticed the T-shirt. Their response was 50 per cent. The group the students had briefly met were also asked if they had noticed the appearance of the Barry Manilow T-shirt. Only 20 per cent had.

We think we're in the spotlight when we're not. And we overestimate the impact of embarrassing moments. The 'spotlight effect' explains why people think their shortcomings and failings are far more noticeable than they actually are. Most of the time, most people don't notice. They're caught up in their own spotlight.

So don't overreact if you commit a gaffe. Others will probably not have noticed, but they will note your exaggerated response to your mistake when you draw attention to it. Don't turn a minor mistake into a major embarrassing episode – for you and for others.

14.4.3   Those Who Matter and Those Who Mind

Be who you are and say what you feel, because those who mind don't matter and those who matter don't mind.

Dr Seuss

Don't worry too much about criticisms from those who 'mind'. In the long run, they might not 'matter'.

Don't be embarrassed. Don't allow any sense of social awkwardness stop you from doing what you want to do.

And if you do get embarrassed, so what? It's a small price to pay if it helps you achieve your goals.

Ask yourself:

• Would it be so bad if I got embarrassed? What would be the consequences?

14.5   Managing Those Moments of Anxiety

We can easily manage if we will only take, each day, the burden appointed to it. But the load will be too heavy for us if we carry yesterday's burden over again today, and then add the burden of the morrow before we are required to bear it.

John Newton

The capacity to imagine – to look into the future and see new possibilities – was probably humanity's greatest evolutionary gain. But it comes at a price. While we can envisage positives, we can also anticipate negatives. And uncontrolled, our imagination creates worry. Instead of motivating us into problem-solving mode, worry becomes counter-productive anxiety and inaction.

You can manage your worries in several ways:

• **Accepting worry as a life fact**. Worry helps prepare you for the future, identifying the challenges you need to overcome to make progress in life. But make sure you balance your worries with positives about your present and future.
• **Controlling your worry time**. Rather than allowing worries to invade every minute of your day, schedule in a 20-minute 'worry session'. Any worries that enter your consciousness outside this time should be written down and saved for review. Try to plan your 'worry time' for the same time each day – but don't make it just before you head for bed.
• **Talking logically to yourself**. If the problem can be solved then why worry? If the problem cannot be solved worrying will do you no good. Treat each worry as a problem to be solved:
  – Translate the worry into a practical problem. How would others define this worry?
  – Think of all the possible solutions to the problem. What has worked for you in the past when faced with a similar worry?

 – Work through the pros and cons of different solutions and choose one that you feel can work for you.
 – Map out the key actions you will undertake to implement the solution.
- **Drawing on others' support**. A problem shared is not always a problem halved. But others – family, friends, colleagues – can be an invaluable resource in helping you overcome life's problems. Don't go it alone when you can call on the experience, insights, and ideas of those who have had similar problems.

14.6   Managing Mistakes as an Indicator of Assertiveness

14.6.1   Mistakes Indicate Progress

Learn from your mistakes quickly. Mistakes are fundamental to learning. If you're not making mistakes, the chances are that you're not learning and you aren't making progress in life. But don't make the mistakes that keep you in the same classroom of life. Pay attention to your experience. Don't dismiss any failure as 'one of these things that could happen to the best of us'. Ask why:

- What did you do?
- What didn't you do?
- What would you do differently faced with a similar situation in future?

   Learn from your successes:

- What worked?
- Why?

Don't assume that the same approach will always work:
- What would you do differently to be even more successful?

   In dentistry mistakes are all too often a team failing, so it is important to discuss both personal and group errors together, learn from them, and incorporate that learning into future audit meetings.

14.6.2   Admit Honest Mistakes

Don't defend the indefensible. If you've made a mistake, say so and say it quickly. Don't overdo explanations of what you did or why you did it. Focus on what you need to do in the future.

   Invariably, it is our response to mistakes rather than the mistake itself that creates the bigger problem. You aren't perfect, so don't put yourself through the mill if and when you do get something wrong. But do find ways to put things right.

14.6.3   Some Mistakes Matter More Than Others

Mistakes are inevitable and are an integral part of your professional development. But some mistakes will destroy your credibility overnight.

Mistakes made in the attempt to implement innovations within your practice are part of the process of learning and are understandable. Mistakes arising out excessive commitment can be forgiven.

However, mistakes of judgement, particularly in the area of personal ethics and morality, will permanently damage your credibility. And if you jeopardise others' reputations, such mistakes won't be overlooked.

14.6.4 Don't Make the Mistake Worse

Deal with your mistakes well. It is your response to your mistakes that makes the difference:

- Don't fail to admit the mistake.
- Don't deny that it ever happened or attempt to cover it up.
- Don't fail to take steps to 'fix' or alleviate the effects of the mistake.
- Don't blame factors outside your control.
- Don't attack other people for their mistakes.

Admit the problem and get on with the task of putting things right. Deception, cover-ups, and attributing blame elsewhere will create a bigger problem in the long run.

14.7 Assertiveness as the Art of the Apology

> *An apology isn't an apology unless you experience a change in heart.*

There is an art to apologising. It isn't:

- The excuse: 'I'm sorry... but...' 'It happened but it wasn't really my fault, something else happened.'
- The denial of intent: 'I'm sorry... I wanted to...' 'My intentions were good, but I'm really a victim of events.'
- Blame: 'I'm sorry... someone else let me down...' 'I did my best but others didn't.'

Apologise and apologise with grace, accepting your responsibility and expressing your commitment to put things right. An effective apology incorporates the following:

- **Recognition**: the apology acknowledges that something has gone wrong and identifies the severity of the problem. The apology empathises with others to see the issue through their eyes and doesn't dismiss what happened as 'one of those things'.
- **Responsibility**: a meaningful apology accepts personal responsibility. Rather than looking around to point the finger of blame, the apology says 'I screwed up'. You might not have personally got things wrong, but accountability requires you to accept responsibility.
- **Remorse**: the apology has empathy with others, seeing the consequences that have resulted from the problem. The apology is a genuine and heartfelt expression of emotion.
- **Restitution**: 'I'm sorry' is easy. More difficult but genuine is 'What do I need to do to put things right?' The apology is a swift response to do whatever needs to be done to restore credibility and reassure others that you are genuine in your commitment.

14.8 How to Project Well

The voice collects and translates your bad physical health, your emotional worries, your personal troubles.

Placido Domingo

It is estimated that when a voice-trained person delivers a speech, the audience retains 83 per cent of the information. In contrast, when an untrained person delivers the same speech, the audience will only retain 45 per cent of the information. People switch off quickly if your voice is boring, monotonous, or expressionless.

14.8.1 The 4 Ps

Pay attention to the 4 Ps to ensure effective public speaking:

- **Pace** should be neither too fast nor too slow. Too fast, and you gabble and undermine your credibility. Too slow, and the audience switches off. Vary the pace, particularly when you express a new point.
- **Pitch** should not be so low you can't be heard, nor so high you sound nervous. Modulate your pitch for emphasis.
- **Pauses** should be built into your speech. Well-timed pauses create suspense to get attention, or can be used as a powerful exclamation mark. Slow down when you want to make a new point.
- **Passion** should indicate your interest and enthusiasm in your topic. If you aren't passionate about the topic, change the topic or avoid public speaking about it.

14.8.2 Voice Tips

There are some things you can do to ensure you project your voice well:

- **Posture**. Stand up straight and tall to allow full lung capacity and airflow.
- **Breathe well**. Practise long and controlled exhales. When you speak, use your breath to punctuate your point. Take a breath at the end of each phrase whether you need to or not. Use that opportunity to pause and let the listeners absorb what you are saying.
- **Articulate**. Try exaggerating your lip movements to reduce mumbling. Practise articulating tongue-twisters and extending and exaggerating vowel sounds.
- **Loosen up** before you begin. Look from side to side. Roll your head in half-circles and roll your shoulders back. Shift your rib cage from side to side. Yawn. Stretch. Touch your toes while completely relaxing your upper body, then slowly stand up.
- **Record** your voice using different ways of speaking. Determine which one is most effective given the nature of the material and the make-up of the audience.

14.9 Fundamentals of Presentations

We're not all natural presenters, but with an understanding of what makes an effective presentation, the desire to have a go, and the willingness to learn from feedback, we can all deliver a credible presentation (or at least one that doesn't damage our reputation).

14.9.1   Avoid Obvious Mistakes

Sometimes failure provides more learning than success. Here are seven reasons why presentations often don't have the impact and influence they should have:

- **Dependence on mechanical aids.** Have a story to tell, don't run through the bullet-point script of a PowerPoint presentation.
- **Failure to research the audience.** Know what matters to those who are listening to you and how to connect to their interests and priorities.
- **Unsupported opinions.** Be provocative and controversial, but don't be opinionated and dogmatic.
- **Wrong facts.** Don't let inaccuracy about specific facts and figures undermine a compelling argument.
- **Lack of audience involvement.** Lectures rarely create action. Engage and interact with your listeners.
- **Speaking in a monotone.** Don't let a boring delivery undermine a compelling argument.
- **Politically incorrect behaviour.** Choose your words well and avoid taking a risk on untested humorous material.

14.9.2   Prepare for Presentations

As Mark Twain said: 'It takes more than three weeks to prepare a good impromptu speech.' Presentations can be high-stakes moments in your professional life, situations with the potential to raise your profile and establish a reputation, or to damage your credibility. Prepare well by:

- **Researching your audience**: know what matters to them and will engage their interest.
- **Rehearsing your speech**: record yourself and listen back to gauge the pace and tone of your delivery.
- **Managing your voice**: project enthusiasm and speak from the heart with conviction.
- **Practising your technique**: get feedback to keep fine-tuning how you construct your presentation content and organise its delivery. Brilliant presenters weren't always brilliant.

14.9.3   Know Your Topic in Detail

Identify the question you want the audience to engage in rather than the answer you want to provide. Anticipate questions. Have the facts at your fingertips.

14.9.4   Speak with Power

Effective communication is not about the number of things you say or how clever or charming you are in saying them. It is about conveying a message that others understand and that changes their way of thinking about your position. You can help ensure this by:

- Saying fewer things, but with conviction and slowly. Be prepared to repeat what you have said, and to follow up with a simple statement of the issues.

- Watching your use of 'you know', 'sort of' and 'maybe'. This kind of vagueness undermines your credibility.
- Avoiding conversational 'clichés', those worn-out phrases that make for a stale and dull presentation.

14.9.5 Simplicity

Staying simple sharpens up presentations. As Aristotle observed: 'It is simplicity that makes the uneducated more effective than the educated when addressing popular audiences.' Keep your presentations simple by having a key idea, an interesting story, challenging findings or statistics, and a compelling logic. And use this simplicity to connect to and interact with your audience.

14.9.6 End Well

A happy exit is better than applause on entrance. Many meetings and presentations begin big and engage the audience. But then the momentum goes and the session fizzles out, leaving the group wondering 'What was that all about?'

Start well to gain your audience's attention, but also make sure your conclusion is memorable. Use your best story, most compelling statistic, and key recommendations to finish well.

Do

14.10   How to Be Assertive

There are six ways to be more assertive:

- **Repetition and the 'broken record'**: firmly repeat your request, particularly when you feel you're not being taken seriously.
- **Fogging**: in the face of criticism, stay calm and agree with those aspects that are fair. By acknowledging where you could have done better and refusing to become upset, you defuse the critic's destructive words. Use phrases like 'you have a point there' and 'some of that is true but. . .'
- **Following DESC scripting**:
  - **D**escribe what seems to happening.
  - **E**xpress how you feel.
  - **S**pecify what you'd like to happen.
  - Then outline the **C**onsequences of what will happen if you don't get your way.
- **Using 'I' language**: be specific in the way you express yourself, saying 'I feel. . .' and 'I intend to. . .' Keep the focus on your desired outcomes.
- **Seeking workable compromises**: when there is a conflict between what you want and what the other person wants, assertiveness is not about dominating to win, it is about negotiating a position that takes both parties' needs into account.
- **Practising the skill**: review your experience and what you have learnt from the exercise.

In a Nutshell: Be Assertive

Why is assertiveness an issue for some people but not others? In our personal and professional lives there will be times when assertiveness is critical to a successful outcome.

In this chapter you will have learnt how to deal assertively with the challenges presented by criticism and how to avoid embarrassment to get critical points across,

You have discovered how to apologise with grace, recognising what has gone wrong, your responsibility, and next steps.

This chapter ended by drawing your attention to some presentation fundamentals to help you communicate well.

Index

Leadership Skills for Dental Professionals: Begin Well to Finish Well, First Edition.
Raman Bedi, Andrew Munro and Mark Keane.
© 2022 John Wiley & Sons Ltd. Published 2022 by John Wiley & Sons Ltd.